Advance Praise

"Kathrin Stauffer, a relational psychotherapist, appreciates that a human body is born equipped to share affections, often without words, in proud and joyful activity with companions. We are not to be left in loneliness, struggling with sad worries or guilt of a Self-out-of-relations. She describes work to support four adults, each experiencing anxiety and shame after a childhood of neglect. This is a lesson in ways to share recovery of healthy pride in systems of companionship, a therapy that is interpersonal, relational, and dyadic. Following advances in the psychology of infancy in the 1960s, the last two decades have brought evidence of human sympathy in relations, from the neuroscience of affections, from proof that consciousness arises in prospective control of form and power in movements, and from evidence that the brain is built for intersubjective sharing of purposes and emotions in expressive activity."

—**Colwyn Trevarthen**, Ph.D., FRSE, Professor (Emeritus) of Child Psychology and Psychobiology, School of Philosophy, Psychology and Language Sciences, The University of Edinburgh

"Kathrin Stauffer provides intelligent, accessible theory along with common-sense interventions to ease frustrations that too often result when attempting work with clients who have been emotionally neglected as children. Carefully chosen, poignant case examples throughout the book illustrate the depth and breadth of these issues. At the core, Stauffer's dedication to her clients shines through and is translated into a book offering the knowledge, insight, sensitivity, and compassion necessary to help these heretofore lost-in-the-cracks clients."

—**Babette Rothschild**, author of *The Body Remembers* and *Revolutionizing Trauma Treatment*

EMOTIONAL NEGLECT
AND THE ADULT IN THERAPY

EMOTIONAL NEGLECT
AND THE ADULT IN THERAPY

Lifelong Consequences
to a Lack of Early Attunement

KATHRIN A. STAUFFER

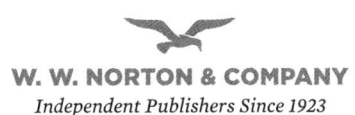

W. W. NORTON & COMPANY

Independent Publishers Since 1923

Note to Readers: Standards of clinical practice and protocol change over time, and no technique or recommendation is guaranteed to be safe or effective in all circumstances. This volume is intended as a general information resource for professionals practicing in the field of psychotherapy and mental health; it is not a substitute for appropriate training, peer review, and/or clinical supervision. Neither the publisher nor the author(s) can guarantee the complete accuracy, efficacy, or appropriateness of any particular recommendation in every respect. As of press time, the URLs displayed in this book link or refer to existing sites. The publisher and author are not responsible for any content that appears on third-party websites.

For information about permission to reproduce selections from this book, write to Permissions, W. W. Norton & Company, Inc., 500 Fifth Avenue, New York, NY 10110

For information about special discounts for bulk purchases, please contact W. W. Norton Special Sales at specialsales@wwnorton.com or 800-233-4830

Manufacturing by Versa Press
Production manager: Katelyn MacKenzie

ISBN: 978-0-393-71441-8

W. W. Norton & Company, Inc., 500 Fifth Avenue, New York, N.Y. 10110
www.wwnorton.com

W. W. Norton & Company Ltd., 15 Carlisle Street, London W1D 3BS

2 3 4 5 6 7 8 9 0

For my father, the original ignored child.

Contents

Introduction   xi

CHAPTER 1

The Experience of Being an Ignored Child   1

CHAPTER 2

Possible Scenarios of Emotional Neglect   35

CHAPTER 3

Psychotherapeutic Theories About Ignored Children   53

CHAPTER 4

Neuroscientific Contributions Toward
Understanding Ignored Children   89

CHAPTER 5

General Principles for Psychotherapy
with Adults Who Were Ignored Children   127

CHAPTER 6

Specific Psychotherapeutic Interventions   161

Concluding Remarks   203

Acknowledgments   215

References   217

Index   229

Introduction

A client presents for psychotherapy with anxiety and stress. They give an impression of struggling with life and finding everything hard work, without having much idea why this is so. They will be very polite, rather shy, and come across as a bit split off from their feelings.

It will be hard for the therapist to get a clear history from this client, who will say things like, "Nothing bad has ever happened to me," or "Everything was fine, and I shouldn't be having problems really." This absence of a narrative to account for their difficulties will be noticeable.

The client will be motivated to work hard in psychotherapy, but typically will be rather lost as to how to do this. They may need quite a lot of direction from the therapist. If the therapist does not give such direction, the therapeutic process will soon feel as if it has run aground and got stuck. The therapist may in that case begin to feel that the client does not really want to get better, and the therapist may give up on them. If the therapist does give direction, the client may follow it with great relief; or they may argue that it is impossible for them to do so. The therapist will probably experience the client as avoidant, defended, lacking spontaneous aliveness, and generally as a person who suppresses their inner life.

Typically this client will be anxious, although the anxiety may not be very noticeable, rather as if the client were at pains to hide their anxiety from others. It may emerge in the course of several sessions just how all-pervasive the anxious feelings are. It will become apparent that the client has poor affect-regulation skills and is split off from their body, and through this from their deeper vitality.

The client will have a tendency to ruminate and worry, especially about their health. They may not have many interpersonal resources and may suffer from social anxiety, shyness, or awkwardness in the company of others, including the therapist. To the discerning therapist it will soon dawn that the client suffers from crippling shame, but it may be rather nebulous what this shame is about, other than not functioning like other people.

Typically, such a client will strongly resist therapeutic change. They may give an impression of having no hope of improvement, or of being too afraid of change, or of not wanting to get better. The therapist may experience this as passive-aggressive behavior or as a sabotaging attack on the therapy. It will take deeply compassionate insight for the therapist to realize that the client has so few resources that they cannot afford to risk losing any, and therefore change has to be negotiated in tiny steps and at a snail's pace.

In the course of therapy, it will gradually emerge that this client suffers from early emotional neglect. I have come to call these clients ignored children, because their history is typically one of being ignored by their caregivers as infants or young children. They may not have been rejected or abused early in their lives; but they were not made to feel welcome, loved, and safe in the world either, and they didn't have their needs met or even seen. Instead they were taken for granted, overlooked, treated like adults from a very young age, or used by their caregivers to help, without receiving any positive attention in return.

What I call emotional neglect is specifically the experience in the first months and years of life up to age about six years of not feeling welcomed, not being seen as a separate person, and not having one's needs met or even perceived by caregivers. In the life of an emotionally neglected child, there is no adult caregiver who is reliably available when the child needs an adult. There is no caregiver to show the child that their presence gives the caregiver joy, no caregiver to look after the child and keep them safe, and no adult caregiver for the child to reach out to for help and support. Instead, ignored children are on their own and have to look after themselves—indeed, often they have to parent not only themselves but also their parents.

In recent years, psychotherapists have learned an enormous amount about abuse in early life and how this affects its victims in later life. Often people who have been neglected are bracketed in with abused people by mental health professionals, but a person with a history of being neglected is different from a person with a history of being abused. Although both a neglected and an abused person are traumatized, the nature of the traumatization of the neglected person is characteristic and distinct from that of an abuse victim. I will elucidate the main characteristics of clients with a history of early emotional neglect in the following chapters.

The main consequence of emotional neglect is that the person will grow up with developmental deficits. This means that the person will be rather like a child trying to live the life of an adult person: they are constantly overstretched, overreaching themselves, having to run to keep up. The traumatization of a neglected person is therefore akin to burnout, because it results from having to do too much with too few resources. As a consequence, the cultivation of new resources in therapy will be of central importance.

In clinical practice we also find that developmental deficits make it extremely difficult to change, because the scarcity of resources means that a person cannot ever risk losing anything that contributes to their habitual functioning. Because of this, psychotherapy with clients who have been emotionally neglected is very slow, and change can only happen in very small increments and by the addition of new resources that don't constitute a threat to old ones.

Other main consequences of early emotional neglect are the experiences of feeling ignored, unwanted, and uncared for. Being ignored is likely to lead to powerful anxiety, because for a very small child it is dangerous to be ignored. Feeling unwanted will almost certainly lead to pervasive and toxic shame. Both the anxiety and the shame will be generalized and persistent in adults who were ignored children, and it will not be easily possible to trace them to specific conflicts within the person.

The experience of being unparented and uncared for will create a person who often feels bewildered by life, as if they had not been taught how to "do" life. This in turn may make situations involving some expression of spontaneity, such as making a choice or being playful, very anxiety-provoking and shame-inducing. It will also create a person who does not expect any help or support from others but takes it for granted that they can only rely on themselves. Individuals with an experience of being unparented may grow up with a powerful longing for others to provide them with direction and clear instructions and for somebody to take responsibility for their lives.

Children who are being neglected by their caregivers are likely to develop very insecure attachment bonds where the child will never make trouble and, indeed, may fear any expression of temperament from another person that looks as if it is putting strain on a relationship. This attachment style (which may very well superficially look avoidant and dismissive) is likely to persist into adulthood.

The available scientific literature suggests strongly that the impact of emotional neglect in early childhood is as great as the impact of emotional abuse in terms of mental and physical health as well as social functioning of adults (for a summary of the literature see Sciarrino, Hernandez, & Davidtz, 2018). One study showed that emotional neglect leaves children with a more reactive amygdala, leading to the assumption that these people will be more prone to anxiety throughout life (Bogdan, Williamson, & Hariri, 2012; De Bellis et al., 2009). Other studies have looked at the children of mothers with postnatal depression and found that these are at severe risk from depression themselves (Murray & Cooper, 1996). Attachment research has pointed for a long time to the lifelong consequences of insecure attachment (Gauthier et al., 1996). Overall, the evidence is growing to suggest that ignored children may be condemned to enormous suffering as adults (Joseph, 1999).

I have had the privilege to work therapeutically with many clients who were ignored children, and I feel that I have learned a lot about their experience and also about how to work therapeutically with them. I have found that many psychotherapists struggle to work with these clients, mainly for two reasons: (1) these are clients who look as though they are quite high functioning but who are in reality much more vulnerable than is visible and (2) the therapeutic process is very slow—unbearably so for some therapists.

Many times, as I have shared some of my therapeutic experience with ignored children, my peers and supervisees have asked me for titles of books that they could read in order to learn more. As a consequence I discovered that early emotional neglect is also a very neglected topic in the literature (Hobbs & Wynne, 2002; Leeds, 2012). Relatively few papers or books explore the treatment of childhood neglect or attempt to develop specific interventions (Allin, Wathen, & MacMillan, 2005; Leeds, 2015; Muller, 2010; Paulsen, 2017). This has led me to write this book, in order to contribute what I know to the field.

This book is written specifically for psychotherapists who work with adults. Psychotherapists who work with children may not find it very useful, because I am not offering any information about child psychotherapy. People who are not psychotherapists may find some interesting and perhaps useful insights into their own inner life, if they were ignored children, or into the inner life of people near them who were ignored children.

My main interest is in the clinical practice of psychotherapy. I originally trained as a body psychotherapist and have since added to my resources more knowledge of psychotherapy in general, as well as some training mostly aimed at trauma treatment that I find useful. My original body psychotherapy training has taught me that therapeutic processes have their own time; even if a process is very slow, we can discern that it is happening if we observe our clients well. Moreover, I find that however slow a process of healing is, once it has reached a certain momentum it cannot easily be stopped.

Because this book is about emotional neglect, I will not say much about physical neglect of children, except to note that there is a large overlap and that especially in families where there are not enough available caregivers and not enough material resources, both physical neglect and emotional neglect may go together (Nikulina & Widom, 2014; Widom et al., 2012). I am aware that past physical neglect will have emotional consequences in the present, and these I will work with.

I will also not say much about child abuse, be it physical, emotional, or sexual. Again, I am aware that there is a large overlap and that many people who present for psychotherapy with a history of abuse also have a history of neglect. Even so, I have deliberately constructed my case examples to be of people who do not have a history of abuse. Abuse is generally easier to spot for therapists, and there is a large body of literature about it. This is not the literature situation for emotional neglect, and my emphasis is on looking at the clinical presentation of neglect as distinct from abuse. Therapists who work with clients with a complex trauma history that includes both abuse and neglect may find some of what I describe here helpful, both in terms of understanding some of the peculiarities of their clients and also in terms of informing their thoughts about what treatments may work well.

I have organized the book to reflect my way of thinking about ignored children. Chapter 1 outlines details of clinical presentations, with an emphasis on the client's subjective experience. Chapter 2 looks at the typical histories and at possible primary scenarios that may result in emotionally neglected children. Chapters 3 and 4 present theoretical models that contribute to the understanding of these clients. I have divided these somewhat arbitrarily into more *psychotherapeutic* and more *neuroscience-derived* theoretical approaches. Chapters 5 and 6 are concerned with the therapy of emotionally neglected clients. Chapter 5 sets out important therapeutic considerations specific to this client group—what I call the relational aspects of working with ignored children. Chapter 6 describes in more detail the particular psychotherapeutic approaches that I have found useful and outlines how I apply these. In my concluding remarks, I will say something about ignored children and their place in the contemporary Western world, where they may struggle to find acceptance and where they may be misunderstood, misconstrued, exploited, or discriminated against.

In order to illustrate the material, I have constructed four clients who represent different facets of adults with a history of emotional neglect who present for therapy. The therapeutic process of these four clients is woven through the book and I hope will make it more readable and more alive.

EMOTIONAL NEGLECT
AND THE ADULT IN THERAPY

CHAPTER 1

The Experience of Being an Ignored Child

Introducing My Four Clients

Mortimer is in his twenties and presents for therapy because he suffers from anxiety. He tells me, "I don't know why I am so anxious all the time, but I've probably been like this all my life. I just seem to have been born without confidence." An only child of two ambitious parents with high-flying business careers, he grew up a shy boy who was labeled "nerdy" at school and at times bullied. In college he flourished a little more and managed to obtain a good degree and also a girlfriend with whom he now lives. Professionally, he feels that he has stagnated since he graduated, finding most jobs difficult and stressful. Socially, he is withdrawn a lot of the time, so that his girlfriend is currently getting more and more frustrated, which distresses him greatly, because he fears she may leave him. He doesn't feel able to say this to her and so he sees no way out of the distress.

His narrative of his own childhood is that he was rather spoiled, as only children often are. He feels he never learned to look after himself and worries that he was a disappointment to his parents. Both parents are still very important people in his life, and he will make large sacrifices to his own comfort in order to accommodate their needs, particularly if his mother needs anything. He emphasizes the gratitude he feels toward his parents for the happy and safe childhood they gave him.

Mortimer is difficult to work with—he is typically anxious coming into the therapy room and finds it hard to get started. If I wait for him to speak, his anxiety quickly increases. He experiences my silence as punitive and as pressure to perform. He feels shamed by many, if not most, of my attempts to mirror back his experience. He struggles to talk about how he feels because he either doesn't feel anything or can't find the words for it. He does not like to speak about his childhood, because it seems ungrateful toward his parents. "Just the thought that I might be unfair toward my parents makes me anxious," he says. He knows of a few things that have happened to him that were not okay, but can't see the point in talking about them over and over again. He also doesn't feel that they were quite bad enough to account for how terrible he feels most of the time. He is too embarrassed to do anything other than sit in his chair and resists movement or bodywork of any kind. In fact, most ways of working in psychotherapy that I have available are not possible for him, and sessions with Mortimer are like being surrounded by closed doors and having more doors slammed shut whenever I try to find an open one. I take this to be what it is like to be inside his mind—a constant scrabbling round for an escape without ever finding one. To me this feels like a terrible torture.

Norman is in his fifties when he comes to therapy, a fairly senior civil servant who has remained single without quite understanding why. He comes because he feels lonely and has bouts of depression that are getting worse. "I'm sure I'm just having a midlife crisis," he says. "But sometimes my life seems so empty I just can't stand it anymore."

Norman lost his mother early in life to a lingering illness. He was cared for by various relatives for a number of years until his father remarried. He then acquired several younger half siblings. He says he always felt like he didn't belong in this family, and he doesn't have much contact with any of them now.

His life is that of a workaholic, and he is used to working long hours and not having much time to himself. In his free time he attends various cultural activities and reads a lot. It is the solitary life of somebody who has trained himself to be alone until he doesn't really have much use for other people anymore.

In therapy, Norman initially attempts to look after me by working hard and diligently. He would like homework and also wants to understand what we are doing and why. He knows that losing his mother early on has been a big trauma in his life, but doesn't know what exactly the impact was and how he could change this. I soon realize that often after sessions he goes home feeling deeply despondent and hopeless and trapped in the way he is, so that coming back the following week seems pointless and unnecessarily stressful. To my question about this, he says, "I know that talking about it all is supposed to make it better, and I like the illusion that I have for a short time, that somebody cares. But then, when I go home, I'm by myself again; and I have time to think about all the things I should not have said, or should have said differently, and I can't stop thinking about all that."

I realize from this statement that every session throws him back into the abandoned place where he had thought that somebody cared, and then they were not there anymore, and he is desperately trying to find out what he needs to do differently in order for them to stay. The little exchange opens the way for a deeper exploration of this and for more understanding on his part.

———

Olivia has a history of unsatisfactory relationships and wants to work on this. She looks like a successful professional, highly intelligent and articulate, and very self-aware. It is a pleasure to have conversations with her, and it takes me quite a while to realize how few and brittle her resources are and how vulnerable she is to stress. It turns out she was given up by her mother soon after her birth and later adopted. She thus grew up with a mother who couldn't have her own children and was full of bitterness because of this. Inevitably, some of this bitterness was felt by Olivia. She tells me that she used to fantasize about her real mother and how lovely it would be to find her, but she never has.

In relationships, she usually assumes that she is not good enough and constantly expects to be abandoned. Mostly this makes her adopt a cautious and even sometimes avoidant stance, while also being quite submissive. Several of her partners have commented on how irritating her habit of apologizing for everything is. On the inside she experiences herself as always just on the verge of becoming clingy. She lives in a world where she is basically unwelcome and cannot take anything for granted, but is forever longing to be welcomed and wanted. A few times in her life she has met somebody who has made her feel more welcome, but the feeling has never lasted, and attempts to get close to such a person have been terrifying for her. Each time this happened it left her with more fear of getting close to others. "I feel as if life is playing a game with me, and as soon as I can even see something I want, it gets snatched out of my reach."

Toward me her avoidance is evident. Although we have regular sessions, talking, sometimes making drawings or paintings, sometimes doing bodywork, I very often feel that Olivia will not let me get close beyond a certain point. Initially I perceive this as rather arrogant and dismissive, until one day we are talking about shame and she suddenly says, "Well, it happens here, too: every time I have kept you at bay I felt that I was being an arrogant bitch and hating myself for it. The fact is of course that I can't let you get close, no matter how hard I try—but I don't understand why not. More reason for shame." Once I understand this heartbreaking reality of her inner world, we can start to explore the distance between us a little more freely.

Pearl is a very exhausted mother of three teenage children and works as an elementary school teacher. She comes to therapy as her relationship with her 15-year-old daughter is deteriorating very badly. She describes the daughter as going wild and engaging in unsafe behavior and at the same time being highly critical and attacking toward her, especially when she expresses her maternal feelings, and this makes her feel like a total failure. She confesses, "I feel so inadequate and so ashamed of not getting on better with my daughter."

Not entirely surprisingly I find that she has often suffered from inconsiderate and bullying colleagues at work. Her main response to criticism seems to be to try harder, and her boundaries are almost nonexistent. "I cannot imagine not responding when somebody needs me!" she exclaims.

The signs of her being ignored as a child are there: she was her mother's first child, and the family anecdote is that her mother gave her back to the midwife when she found that she had given birth to a girl. Several years later, Pearl acquired a younger brother, the much-prized heir of the family. Later still, a second little brother arrived who was so sweet that he became everybody's favorite. Pearl's role in growing up mostly seemed to be to look after these younger brothers.

Pearl has always been very compliant and tried hard to be "good." She does the same in therapy, rather idealizing me and often emphasizing how helpful the therapy is for her. At the same time, she consistently bats off any attempts of mine to suggest even small ways in which she could look after herself better and shift the balance between her care for others and her care for herself a little more toward herself. There are always compelling reasons that she just has to look after somebody else first right now! One day, I try to move the discussion away from the practical question she happens to be talking about to the more general question of why it would be a good idea for her to look after herself better. I can immediately see her anxiety shooting up into near panic. Unfortunately, she doesn't have the confidence to fend off what to her feels like my attempt to put pressure on her, and if I hadn't seen the panic in her eyes, I might have missed the opportunity. Once I've shared my observation that I seem to have said the wrong thing, we can actually start to look at the issues that have been provoked. "I felt like you were asking me to stop caring for my children, and I didn't think I could do that. It's like you wanted me to be a different person. I've always tried so hard to be kind and caring, and I wouldn't want to be any other. If I started to look out for myself more, I would surely end up ignoring and neglecting my children, and that thought really panics me," she explains. I begin to see how the attacks from her daughter, whom she tries so hard to care for, feel to her like attacks on a coping strategy she has worked hard to develop and needs very badly. This is what makes her daughter's attacks so provocative for her.

What my four clients have in common is the history of emotional neglect in early childhood. What distinguishes them are different ways of coping with their early emotional neglect. While I recognize that there is a lot of overlap between abuse and neglect, I have deliberately chosen clients who do not have a history of abuse. This is because emotional neglect leaves people struggling in particular ways that deserve addressing separately, and this is what I am setting out to do in this book.

I will continue the stories of my four clients' therapy as and when it seems appropriate throughout the book.

Understanding the Inner World of Emotionally Neglected People

When children are born, they have just experienced the end of all life as they knew it previously, which took place in their mother's womb. Miraculously, they don't respond to this by clinging to intrauterine life and withdrawing from the world—on the contrary, they are fully oriented to getting on with life and making themselves at home in the newly gained world. Newly born babies are generally wide awake and seek contact with whoever is there to receive them. Establishing eye contact with a loving mother or other caregiver is as important as taking the first breath, learning how to take in nourishment, or getting used to gravity. This eye contact gives the newly born child a sense of being welcomed with joy and love in the world. The necessity of being welcomed in this way continues for the first months of a child's life, and attempts to seek that welcome may continue for much longer if the child's welcome is doubtful.

Being welcomed into the world means getting a first, all-important feeling of being loved that can sustain a person through the rest of their life. Most people intuitively know that it is important and life-giving to be welcomed and loved and to see delight reflected in the eyes of others. Research into mothers and infants has caught up with intuition since the middle of the 20th century and now demonstrates clearly just how important it is for a child to have responsive, interactive, and affectionate caregivers who are capable of seeing the child for who they are and who are concerned for the child's well-being. It can be shown that the very growth of connections in the brain depends on contact with such caregivers and on the little glances between the baby and their caregivers, the small rhythmical exchanges that sound like nonsense to an observer, the moments of intimacy and shared pleasure.

It is a terrible thing for a baby to meet with disgust, anger, or abuse from its caregivers. However, it is an equally terrible thing for a child to be ignored, to meet with indifference with nothing. From benevolent and responsive caregivers, children can learn that they are loved and that they are good people. They can learn that it is worthwhile to communicate their needs and wishes to the world and to protest when they are uncomfortable. They can learn that other people are where safety is and that making contact can give them good feelings. If caregivers ignore babies, babies may not have a chance of learning any of this. Instead they may come to live in a world that is cold and indifferent, that they cannot influence and that doesn't give them anything good. This engenders a lot of fear in ignored children. Fear is a realistic response for a small child in this situation, because a small child who is not cared for can easily die. When the child's upbringing continues in the same way, the fear may also continue. Most people who live with this fear learn to numb it, to switch off from it, so that they no longer perceive it and are no longer crippled by it. However, the fear continues to be present in the physical body and can manifest in different ways: as anxiety with no particular content, as physical tension or illness, as shyness, as phobias, as a feeling of being easily overwhelmed from being with other people, as avoidance of social and intimate relationships, or just as a feeling of stress.

The numbing of fear, together with inadequate contact in early life, often has the consequence that all feelings become hard to perceive. The person may live in a fog of unspecific emotion for which they have no words and that they don't know how to express or how to regulate. The only salvation appears to be thought, and so we may be faced with an individual who appears to be "stuck in their head" and not in contact with their feelings. Attempts to bring the person more into contact with feelings may not work at all because they only increase the fear and make everything worse. In fact, the person is not suffering from too little emotion, but from too much—too much fear, specifically—and this cannot be processed or reassured because the blueprints for understanding and being reassured are simply not there. Over time it may be possible to learn such ways of managing, but it will take a long time.

If the person does not understand what happened to them at the beginning of their life, they may never understand their current experience of themselves and other people. They may feel depressed on and off for most of their life. They may find the world a terrifying and hostile place that can only be survived with constant, very great effort.

It is typical of a neglected person that, whatever is not right in their life, there is often no narrative to account for its origin, in the way that a person who has suffered abuse (or a marked loss or a similar event) will have a narrative of, "This happened and it affected me in a certain way, and that's the reason that I am as I am now." A person who has been neglected may not have such a narrative but instead may be left to feel that they are just odd. They may in the past have been blamed for being odd and not responding "like a normal person." Usually they feel dreadfully ashamed of how they are.

When such ignored children present for therapy in adult life, they will give an impression of deeply traumatized individuals, but they may not have a history of traumatic events in their lives. In my experience there are subtle differences in the presentation between abused and neglected clients, although they overlap considerably (and indeed many neglected children also suffer maltreatment or abuse of some kind). There will be few palpable episodes of hyperarousal during therapy sessions. The feel of therapy sessions will be boring rather than scary or dramatic, frozen rather than overheated, as if the absence of something vital comes right into the therapy room. Often there will be a pervasive sense of a thoroughly numbed person, a person who seems to live in a fog, perhaps all the time. Connecting feelings and words may well be very difficult or impossible in this state. The absence of words may also mean that understanding is elusive. There may be little clues as to the presence of a lot of fear: the person may say they are anxious, or they may exhibit a degree of compulsiveness, and certainly their self-esteem will be extremely low—as if they are not allowed to take up space in the world. They may also be extremely anxious to take care of everybody else, including their therapist, in an effort to avoid causing trouble or drawing attention to themselves. They may suffer from physical illness a lot, or from so-called psychosomatic conditions. Usually they offer powerful resistance to therapy. This may take the form of finding good reasons that things will not work; or it may take the form of being very polite and good but maintaining a distance; or it may take the form of accusing themselves of being hopeless. Therapists who attempt to challenge these forms of resistance will find that the challenges don't improve the situation and may make it much worse. If they are observant, they may realize that much of their client's resistance is motivated by fear, or by shame, or by both—and that challenges make both emotions worse and therefore can't work.

The key to understanding how all of these people function lies in appreciating just how few resources they have that they can rely on. Often this is true of both internal and external resources. Everything that contributes to making life good for most of us is terribly precarious and thin on the ground. Relationships have a tenuous and fragile quality and mirror the tenuous and fragile attachments that these people formed with their early caregivers. What little they have can easily be taken away, and indeed such experiences of having something of vital importance taken away often form terrible and traumatic memories. Every loss is huge because there is so little in the first place, so every resource that is present acquires tremendous importance. Nothing can be spared. Every tiny loss threatens their safety. Safety is their primary concern, and they will be incredibly "good," compliant children and equally compliant adults if it earns them safety.

Neglected children may exist in a frozen world, where any movement they make can threaten their fragile safety, and where it is best to make themselves small and stay still and try to keep life on an even keel. Movement, exuberance, reaching for more, and being big, spontaneous, or impulsive are all highly dangerous to neglected children, however much they might want to do, and be, all these things—and envy people who have them available. It is easy to see that this attitude they take up intuitively does nothing in the longer run to improve their lives, but ends up contributing to their impoverished minds through impoverished lives.

For many ignored children, seeing a psychotherapist is a dangerous adventure into trying to change what can probably not be changed and thus risking severe disappointment. However, if they can establish sufficient safety in the therapy room, they often learn to make very good use of therapy, and the sameness of regular appointments, dogged work with modest results, and the slow pace of change typical of in-depth, open-ended psychotherapy may suit ignored children very well.

The nature of the highly insecure attachments that ignored children form implies that it is very difficult for them to let their therapists know what is really happening inside. They are often desperate to convey the impression that everything is fine, and they can come across as quite ambivalent or dismissive toward the therapy. They may also take a long time to dare to protest when something is not okay: placating a caregiver will often be second nature and will be privileged very clearly over self-expression, well-being, or happiness.

Ways to Cope

In the following I will show some of the ways in which ignored children cope, emphasizing different coping strategies for different individuals. I find that most ignored children utilize most, if not all, of these coping strategies but to different extents, and most have a bias toward one or two of them, thus appearing different on the surface while on a deeper level having a lot in common.

One way that ignored children try to cope with the perceived fragility of their attachment bonds is to become extremely sensitive to the mood of others in an effort to preserve what little closeness and safety they have. Sadly, it does not appear to be possible for such small children to be so focused on another without losing awareness of themselves. By the time they are adults, they may come across as very "merged" people, people with extremely weak boundaries and, often, an uncertain identity. They are typically very accommodating and compliant. They will be astute observers of others but may themselves be quite difficult for others to read. They may find reading themselves, their feelings, and moods difficult or impossible, so that the impression is created that they have sacrificed themselves for another person. We can form an image of a small child who is desperately trying to figure out the mood of their caregivers in an effort to make life a little more comfortable, and who has to do this at the cost of their own well-being.

Mostly these ignored children live in a very lonely world, where nobody is on their side, nobody understands, and nobody can make it better. Getting used to this deep loneliness and finding little crumbs of safety and predictability in their environment is an important coping strategy for them. If they present for psychotherapy, it means that a part of them is still alive to the hope that this could change—as if they still remember that other people are the solution, despite their everyday experience that others are the problem.

Because they didn't have a grown-up helping them to regulate their feelings as infants, they may never become very good at it and may therefore be rather preoccupied with seeking safety, stability, and calm in all areas of life and often to the exclusion of any other goal. They will have little or no notion of their own capacity for creating safety for themselves. It is quite typical to hear stories of the terrible price they pay for the little safety that they are able to earn in relationships. Because they start from such a high level of internal stress, they will be extremely vulnerable to the stress of coping with external demands and, because of this, may find that any kind of worldly success is beyond them.

Making themselves small and trying to fade into the background is one way that ignored children may try to cope with both their vulnerability to stress and their uncertain welcome. In adulthood, this means that they will be shy and quiet and show signs of low self-esteem, such as being compliant, diligent, and overly adapted. Their physical presentation may well be unobtrusive, so that they tend to fade into the background. If they manage to form an intimate relationship, they will never rock the boat and may defer to the partner. Sometimes we find that they try to get some of the love and care they need by literally being rather childlike and seeing others as much more grown-up than themselves. They may also feel that they are quite dependent on others and don't cope well with standing on their own feet, to the point where they submerge their own identity in that of their partner. In therapy they are likely to present with issues related to stress and anxiety and also issues around relationship breakups.

Mortimer is my example for this type of coping style. He makes himself small in every possible way and looks as if he is trying to minimize the amount of space he takes up in the world. He also embodies a person on the knife's edge of fearing other people, while at the same time hoping for good things from them, that can be felt in the therapy room: while he is avoidant in most respects, he also never misses a session and is usually at the door a few minutes before the appointed time.

Mortimer is incredibly alert to the moods of important people around him and, when busy attempting to read another person, loses the ability of being in contact with himself and knowing how he feels. His interpersonal boundaries are poor because of that, and in the early stages of therapy, it is very hard for him to stand his ground in any way.

He also tells me repeatedly how much he dislikes drawing attention to himself or standing out. The feeling of being exposed and scrutinized that comes with being looked at is terrifying for him and makes him want to die of shame.

Others may, at a very early age, decide to not need anything since needing something and not getting it is such a painful experience. These people will aim to be self-reliant and independent and in adulthood may become loners who don't appear to miss human contact much and perhaps don't have much use for other people. If others try to reach out to them and make contact, they may avoid responding because they feel burdened by the demands of such contact. They have been described as "hunkered down" (Shapiro, 2009), which gives a very good sense of how they live their lives. They may not present for therapy at all, but if they do it is likely to be because they feel depressed or aimless or have a longing for more contact than they are currently having. Physical symptoms or illness may also be a trigger to get these clients into therapy.

Norman is my example of this, the depressed and lonely client. He illustrates how numbing himself against the pain has brought with it a numbing against all feelings, including joyful ones. All he is left with is the hole inside—a truly formidable price to pay for coping. In him, the longing for contact is much more strongly defended against than the fear of others, presumably as a result of the very traumatic loss early in life. In a sense he is farther away from health than Mortimer because he has taught himself to be so resigned and to no longer strive or even yearn for what he wants.

In other ways, Norman's way to cope is more successful than Mortimer's: for a lot of the time, Norman does not suffer and can thus live in a belief that he has "sorted his problems out." As long as he can keep his depression and loneliness at bay, his way of coping represents quite a successful adaptation. He is also clearly managing to have a measure of success professionally and has acquired the image and reputation of somebody who functions well in the world. As a result of this, it is much harder for him to understand what has gone wrong, and it takes time for his therapist to appreciate just how fragile Norman is behind his stoic facade.

Many ignored children try their best just to be normal. If they are intelligent and observant to begin with, they may well succeed in looking like everyone else. It may not be apparent to them or anyone else that inside they are much more anxious and insecure than their peers and often very crippled by shame about every aspect of themselves. They may eventually seek therapy because a crisis makes it clear to them that they lack something, that there is a hole inside somewhere. They will typically be suffering from low self-esteem or from being overly sensitive or from burning out. In therapy such people often get the wrong treatment because therapists see a high-functioning person and expect them to change rapidly in accordance with this. Therapists may also feel that it is possible to challenge these clients in ways that are devastatingly shaming for them and don't produce any therapeutic result.

Olivia is my example of this coping style, and I am bringing in the topic of shame right from the start because it is so central to her: the shame that stems from really not understanding why she is not "normal" and can't "just get on with it" in the way that other people do. This type of person is, in quite subtle ways, different from a person who has not been emotionally neglected, and it may require some alertness on the part of the therapist to spot it. The presence of a lot of shame may be the first clue to the real history of these clients.

From Olivia, I gain an impression of a carefully balanced and contrived life, in which everything needs to be just so, and every resource has been utilized to maximum capacity. When she talks of her everyday life, it is quite easy to feel the brittleness of the superficial presentation, as well as the amount of effort that goes into maintaining it, and the terrible distress that lies just under the surface.

Yet others learn from a very early age to vicariously gratify some of their needs by looking after others. These may turn into the compulsive caregivers that become members of the caring profession. They may then present for therapy because they burn out with the care for others or when they become angry and resentful with giving too much and not receiving enough.

I have chosen Pearl to represent this coping style. Characteristic of Pearl is that her self-sacrifice does not cover up for resentment and guilt as much as for fear and panic. There may be a hunger for power and control there, but the aim is relational security rather than the pleasure of being powerful. Her solution to the dilemma between fearing others and wanting good things from them is to "delegate" the reaching out to others that she gives care to, while she herself remains on the side of self-reliance and staying clear of her own disappointment.

Yet underneath it her sense of being unwanted or superfluous has never gone away. Rather, it forms a basis of insecurity that can be seen in all domains of her life. Her self-esteem is very low, her boundaries are weak, her anxiety in response to conflicts and dramatic scenes is extremely high, and it invariably takes a very long time for her to recover from an unpleasant exchange with others. The "I'm not good enough" narrative is ubiquitous and distresses her greatly almost every moment of her life.

I have set out four *types* or *coping styles* of ignored children here, based on the observation that most individuals favor particular coping strategies over others. The order is roughly one of increasing adaptiveness of the favored coping style, but I am not intending to suggest that there is otherwise any deep meaning to these types. Rather they are chosen to help therapists recognize that emotionally neglected clients can present in a range of different ways.

The Burden of Shame

I feel it is very important to understand the central role that shame plays in the lives of ignored children. Most people feel that underneath the socially acceptable facade that they present to the world is a person they are ashamed to show to some extent. This person may be weak, vulnerable, greedy, stupid, selfish, arrogant, full of rage, disgusting, needy, impulsive, or in some other way faulty and shameful. Most people learn to live with this and learn that they will not die of shame if others get glimpses of this inner person. They may find that in order to create intimacy, it is a good thing to trust another person to see it.

To ignored children, this shame is catastrophic, overwhelming, and all-consuming. The specific characteristics that an ignored child will be ashamed of can vary and presumably reflect the attitude of their primary caregiver. An ignored child may feel that they are disgusting, or greedy, or just "wrong"—deep down, lacking in some essential human quality. Their shame will have an all-pervasive quality, as if the person's identity and their very soul is shameful.

They will almost certainly attach more shame to the fact that they cannot entirely hide their shameful selves. It feels shameful to be anxious and insecure. It feels shameful not to like boisterous and rough-and-tumble games with other children. It feels shameful to find that they don't enjoy going to clubs and large parties in the same way others do. It feels shameful to be inhibited and socially awkward and unable to make friends easily. It feels shameful to merit the label "introverted" or "avoidant."

And in addition to that, it feels shameful not to be able to just change all this. Ignored children typically live with a sense of constantly letting themselves down and having no one but themselves to blame for their misfortunes. From the list of things that ignored children are ashamed of, it becomes clear that there are here several layers of shame on top of each other, and all of them consist of deeply toxic and indigestible shame.

I have flagged how ashamed Olivia feels of her inability to let me get close to her. This is only the tip of her shame. Underneath there is a layer of shame for apologizing, which stems from the interactions with her partner and which links to the shame about not being like everybody else. There is another layer of shame connected to being inadequate, and underneath all of this is the shame about not being wanted. There is even an echo of the shame that her mother must have felt for getting pregnant without being in a stable relationship with the father of the child.

Mortimer also feels shame a lot. His is more linked to being a disappointment to his parents and being a failure in the world. However, because he is secretly rather ambitious, he feels strongly humiliated by the therapy, by "having to be in therapy," and by most of my interventions that seem to suggest some shortcoming of his or other. His thought, "I should have worked all of this out for myself a long time ago," keeps filling him with shame and is a serious obstacle to his therapeutic progress. It also means that we need to spend time disentangling his healthy and growth-oriented ambition from his shame and his envy of others.

I have written already about Pearl, who feels constantly ashamed of her own shortcomings and her inability to be a more perfect caregiver. Moreover, she is caught in a dilemma in which both sides create shame: not looking after herself adequately is a matter of shame and a flaw to her mind, but looking after herself better carries the shame of being seen as selfish and uncaring. Loosening the stranglehold of this dilemma turns out to be a key component of our therapeutic process, but the shame goes one step further: she also thinks that if she were a more adequate person, she would be able to solve this dilemma by being able to satisfy both demands, and this is an additional cause for shame.

Norman seems the least shame-bound client of the four. His solution, a lifestyle in which he avoids contact with others a lot, has freed him from much of the necessity of feeling ashamed. His confession to me that he ruminates on sessions afterwards in a way that feels unpleasant makes me think that the shame is not far away and that, in isolating himself as he does, he is paying a high price for this relative absence of shame. The course of Norman's therapeutic process confirms this assumption.

Ignored children live in a world where they are always at risk of being criticized and shamed by others. They may well have experienced this in their lives. They may have been bullied or have had overly critical parents, teachers, or other authority figures. Often they will find their way into relationships with equally critical or abusive partners. Even when nobody is criticizing, and when they are living in relatively supportive environments, the fear of the shame will remain a powerful force, inhibiting much movement in their lives. Indeed, it may feel to a person who was an ignored child that it is only their own internal criticism that ensures they remain perceived as a good person and therefore remain safe. We can assume that this habit of self-criticism gives us a window to the internal world of a very small child indeed, who has to construct an internal parent to keep safe. Such a precocious internal parent would appear to be almost inevitably harsh and critical to an extreme degree.

In order to forestall critical and shaming attacks from outside, ignored children will spend an extraordinary amount of time and energy criticizing themselves and scrutinizing their expressions and behavior for potential openings for a critical detractor. As a result, they may well present in therapy feeling that it is this tendency to be terribly critical of themselves that is the problem: being self-critical creates insecurity, lack of self-esteem, low performance, shyness, and so on. They may attempt to rectify matters by seeking cognitive therapies that are good at addressing such self-criticism and low self-esteem, but they will typically find that this does not improve their lives. Therapeutic approaches that are based on an ability of the person to change at will are almost certain not to succeed with ignored children. Because the self-criticism is so necessary for the safety of the person, stopping it is not possible—but usually the person does not know that. So they will simply fail to do what the therapist expects of them, and this will add another layer of shame to the big load of it that they already have to carry around.

Alternatively, clients who are submerged in the necessity of forestalling all external criticism may feel they are successful when they no longer experience external attacks. They may see this as a sign that they have perfected the defense of constantly scrutinizing themselves and their actions and are now able to present a perfect—criticism-proof—result to the world. These clients may then not understand why their lives are such hard work and why they are so exhausted most of the time, failing to see that the solution to suffering from self-criticism is not to be perfect, but to be kind to oneself. Either way, the fact that adults who were ignored children continue to expect shaming and destructive criticism from the world is testimony to the degree to which they are left traumatized by their experiences of early neglect.

The obstacle that shame presents for the psychotherapy of clients who were ignored children is formidable. It is probably safe to assume that every therapeutic intervention, every piece of reflection or mirroring by the therapist, is heard as criticism revealing a shortcoming on the part of the client and will therefore elicit more shame. I do not think there is an easy way around this—an easy way to avoid this almost inseparable intertwining of therapy and humiliation—because people who feel this type of shame are both desperate to be told that they are fine and there is nothing wrong with them (which would relieve the shame but leave them in an unsafe position) and also to be made better and to be helped to at least understand what is wrong (which exacerbates the shame but may lead to more safety). Experience suggests that therapy with ignored children typically takes place in a very narrow space where therapy has a slight edge over shame and that clients have to bear a lot of feeling shamed without walking out on therapy.

In my work with clients who were ignored children, I have always found that they appear to be attached to their inner critic, no matter how savage. This observation confirms my understanding that their shame, and its resulting inner critic, is the only internal caregiver ignored children have available to them. This is one of the insights into the lives of ignored children that breaks my heart, every time. The attachment to the inner critic is one of the factors that makes the therapeutic process with ignored children slow and therefore creates a lot of impatience and frustration in therapists. On the other hand, the recognition that the internal critic is a clumsy attempt at creating an internal parent (by a very little person who doesn't have the knowledge or the skills to create a more sophisticated one) often helps therapists out of this enactment. This recognition also makes the internal critic less formidable and less threatening and allows for more possibility of relating to them in a way that is not characterized only by fear and loathing. It may allow clients to find a more compassionate attitude both toward this clumsy internal parent and also toward the little person who was so unparented that they had to create their own parent at such an early age.

As every therapist knows, parts of the personality that cannot be owned are nearly impossible to change. As soon as some form of truce or peace with them can be reached, there is hope of growing and improving mental well-being. So it is with shame. Once clients stop being terrified, disgusted, or ashamed of their shame, it becomes a phenomenon that can be named, talked about, walked around, and looked at from all sides. Then the scene is set for the client to bring their shame into the contact with the therapist. Shame cannot be discharged in the same way that anger or grief can, through cathartic expression, but it will gradually dissipate when it is brought into contact with another person who does not judge but accepts. This sounds easy, but is not, because it is counterintuitive: a person who feels ashamed intuitively wants to hide their shame and its cause. Therefore, the therapy of disclosing the shame to another person takes tremendous courage for every little bit of shame that gets brought into the contact.

Consequences of Developmental Deficits in the Psychotherapy

One of the most obvious characteristics of clients who were ignored children is that they will appear to resist therapeutic change very strongly. Shame accounts for part of this, as I have attempted to show in the preceding section. In the following section I will attempt to outline other contributing factors.

Children who are being ignored soon learn to look after themselves. Learning what there is to learn for themselves is a part of this enforced autonomy, the result of caregivers who don't provide for the needs of their children. For many ignored children, this works really well on an intellectual level. Typically, ignored children are bright and learn at an early age to use their intellect in order to work out how to cope with life (including how to deal with the relentless internal criticism that helps them preempt and to some extent avoid shaming attacks). They may enjoy how bright they are and develop intellectually in great leaps and bounds. How to be with one's own feelings and emotions, on the other hand, is much harder to learn by oneself, because on the whole this learning happens in contact with other people. Indeed, it could be argued that some of the shame that emotionally neglected people feel is the result of developing ways to manage their own feelings that have not been learned in contact with others and thus acquire a secretive quality that feels shameful.

We learn how to handle our feelings and emotions very early in life, before we learn language and conscious thinking. By the time we become able to make use of verbally spoken or written information, this development is already internalized so firmly that it feels as if it is part of who we are. Moreover, any skill that involves feelings requires the person to be in contact with their own body sensations, because feelings and emotions are inextricably linked to the physical body and its processes. Ignored children who have learned to numb their fears are typically not in good contact with their own bodies, thus further hindering their own emotional development.

Ignored children are quite likely to grow up with large deficits in their emotional development. One of the consequences of developmental deficits is that the person will have to hold on very tightly to what they do have and will be extremely fearful of anything that risks even a small loss. Such a person will then come across as very risk-averse or as very stubbornly resisting change.

Sometimes therapists of clients who so stubbornly resist change attempt to interpret this resistance to the client and to challenge them into giving it up. In my experience this almost never works. The person is so genuinely terrified of what will happen if they change that such challenges inevitably frighten and shame them further. For such an intervention to work, there needs to be a fairly solid ego that integrates to a degree their "feeling" (and perhaps younger) self and their "thinking" (and perhaps more adult) self, so that the here-and-now thought can serve as a container for the primitive fear. In ignored children the connection between these two parts of the person is tenuous and not very permeable, or it is characterized by powerful hostility. There will not be a solid enough basis of thought, supported by feeling, that could contain these fears. Figuratively speaking, there will not be an inner grown-up inside who can take the inner child by the hand and look after the child in the transition.

Many ignored children exist in a state of internal poverty. They live on extremely few resources and feel that there is almost nothing good in their lives. They have few or no friends, perhaps only one or two people who are even a little close. They may give an impression of putting all their eggs in one basket and depending heavily on a very small number of resources. There may be a belief that it would not be safe to augment the number of good things in their lives—they may not deserve the good things, or the danger of losing any of the good things may be too appallingly big, or they may feel unbearably exposed and at risk from having the good things taken away or spoiled by hostile and envious people nearby. Sometimes this fear is so great that the person gets more anxious and appears to be getting worse when there is some therapeutic progress and new resources become available.

Moreover, this internal poverty often connects to a sense that the world is full of impossible demands and that the person is utterly unable to meet these demands. Instead of experiencing opportunities for learning as motivational and as a challenge to be risen to, such opportunities turn into mountains that the person completely lacks the wherewithal to tackle, and they therefore collapse into resignation and more shame. Of course, therapy can also seem such an impossible demand, and therapists need to be aware of the necessity of keeping challenges small enough so that the person can easily meet them. In turn this makes the therapeutic process slow, and progress may seem infinitesimal. It may be important to see, not so much the overall progress the client is able to make, as the success of the strategy of finding small challenges that the client can meet and so build up some *motivational muscle* in preparation for larger challenges ahead.

Mortimer tells me one day that he would like to be challenged more by me. It seems to him that the therapy would go faster if he needed to stretch himself a bit more and not get "spoiled" by me as he believes his mother spoiled him. I get the impression that this request comes from a superego point of view that lacks empathy for the small boy who grew up in a bewildering, cold, and empty world that didn't seem to have a place for him. I have already come across Mortimer's tendency to create unrealistic challenges for himself, born more out of a wish that he could meet them than out of an embodied knowledge of himself and his capabilities.

I start a conversation with him about his relationship with

challenges and say that while I understand his wish to get better more speedily, I would want to be reasonably sure that he can successfully cope with a challenge so that he can experience some satisfaction in successfully meeting it. This is because a feeling of success is an important therapeutic agent. At first, he sees this as humiliating and belittling and starts to argue with me that "rigging" the challenge would spoil the success. We end up having a long conversation about this question: Can he allow himself to have a good feeling of having met a challenge without having to spoil it for himself? He begins to see that he actually does have a choice about this and that not spoiling the feeling of success is a good challenge to set himself.

There is another therapeutic consideration here. Many psycho-therapeutic theories assume that anxious clients suffer from internal conflicts—that is, conflicts between their spontaneous impulses and the more reflective, ego-based part of the personality—and that once these conflicts are named and explored in a relational context, clients can get better. However, clients with large developmental deficits may have anxieties that simply are not based on such internal conflicts; or there may be internal conflicts, but when we start to explore these, we quickly find that they cannot shift because there are not enough inter-nal resources available to allow a movement of what is experienced as an extremely precarious balance. Most classical psychotherapeutic interventions were created for clients caught in a conflict, and they work poorly on clients where this is not the case. We are badly in need of novel therapeutic approaches that work more effectively for people who are not caught in internal conflicts, but simply do not feel safe in the world.

There may be other reasons present for therapy to be very slow, or even for the observation that clients are apparently unable to sustain getting better and get worse again when progress has been made in therapy (this phenomenon has also been called negative therapeutic reaction [Freud, 1962]). In my experience there are often hostile, envious, or extremely deprived elements in the client's early life, such as a mother who felt herself to be so impoverished that any attention she gave to her child represented a deprivation for herself, thus setting up a terrible competition between the two. Here we have another version of the knot between conflict and deficit, this time shared between mother and child: there is not enough psychological good (attention or love) to go around, which is a deficit. Because both mother and child experience taking any good that they get as taking it away from the other, they will both be in a conflict about having it. In that case the conflict maintains the deficit, and in turn the deficit maintains the conflict.

I have already mentioned the severe dilemma in which Pearl finds herself. She turns out to have had a mother who was very preoccupied with her own unhappy marriage and her many unmet needs, who reacted to having a baby with envy of the loving care she had to give this baby. From her later childhood, Pearl remembers comments like, "I don't see why you should have it better than I had it," or "You don't know what real suffering is such as I have experienced," or "If I give you X, you will only become spoiled." Pearl agrees with me that these are all statements that come from feelings of envy. Recalling such memories helps Pearl start to make progress, because it allows her to develop an understanding of the reasons that she finds it so hard to have good things for herself.

Clients who were ignored children describe all sorts of ways in which being ignored has affected them throughout life. One of the common experiences, and one relevant for therapy, is a lack of expectation that the world will help them meet their needs or manage their feelings. There simply isn't a blueprint for such experiences: for example, when child says, "I'm frightened," and a grown-up will be there and say, "Don't worry, I will make sure nothing can harm you." Instead, for an ignored child either there is no grown-up there, the grown-up is too preoccupied with themselves to be available for the child, they don't understand what the child is saying, they are ignorant of what a child needs, they don't feel that the child deserves any help, or they get so frightened themselves by the child's fear that the child ends up having to reassure them. Whichever version of events a person has experienced, it makes reaching out for help or support not a good idea. The result is another contributing factor to slow progress in therapy.

It is part of the human condition that in order to grow, we often have to make a sacrifice and relinquish our previous habits and ways of being so we can find new and more mature ways. For ignored children it may not be possible to undergo this kind of development, because relinquishing anything may not be an option: it may catapult them into the uncontainable terror of total loss, total annihilation. In therapy this means that challenge of any kind is not usually an effective way of working, and we have to do a great deal of building of new resources before we can even think about dismantling any habitual ways of functioning, however maladaptive they may be. Many clients and therapists experience this as a real fear of getting better. Sometimes people create a *secondary gain* narrative around this fear of change. I find it helpful to take this fear seriously and address it as a fear of losing the very precarious hold the person has on whatever they may need to let go of. In developmental terms, we cannot let go of something before we have had it, before we have taken ownership of it, enjoyed it, and taken it for granted—it is only after this that we can let go. If we never establish a firm hold on a developmental stage, we risk remaining forever just on the edges of it, but never able to fully engage with it, and also never able to relinquish it. For some ignored children, this describes the relationship that they have with life.

Compulsive Caregiving

Compulsive caregiving is one of the most adaptive ways of coping with being ignored, and I am therefore giving it a separate section.

For ignored children whose needs are not being met by the outside world, and who have no expectation of this happening, it is an extremely ingenious coping strategy to care for others. First of all, it may cause a preoccupied, depressed, or otherwise emotionally unavailable mother to become friendlier and more affectionate if the child can meet some of her needs or at least adjust their behavior to minimize troubling Mother. Second, an ability to care for others gives the child a little power and a little sense of their own goodness. They won't feel quite so small and insubstantial if they can give something to another and thus have the power of making someone else better. Third, the child may experience vicariously how happy the looked-after person now feels, and while this is not exactly the same as feeling happy oneself, it can come a close second. Finally, caregiving is a way of doing something better than what has been done to the child: knowing the pain of being ignored, they will not do the same to another human being. This last motivation may be present unconsciously only but can be extremely powerful.

Internally, looking after others takes the child away from their own lack and the hollowness that is always there. The child can have an experience of fullness and abundance instead, even if they experience that they are not really able to receive any of this abundance for themselves but can only give it to others. This has the added advantage of making the child feel altruistic and a good person; potentially it also makes the child feel needed and useful, which for many is next best to feeling loved. The pain will not disappear, but it will be dulled, and a successful ignored child can build an identity as someone who is indispensable to others, which may earn them a right to be here and a purpose in life. This coping mechanism allows ignored children to partake in many of life's experiences so that they can feel more part of the human race and not so isolated. It may well satisfy their social needs and some of their attachment needs.

Pearl is the prime example of this coping style. It is characteristic that she doesn't actually see her compulsive caretaking as the problem that needs addressing in therapy, but rather the attacks on it that she has suffered. This is also what creates the burnout—she can no longer sustain a coping style that has become a battle to keep going. Yet as it collapses, she feels she has nothing else and nowhere to turn. Her very identity seems threatened. She is indeed in a profound crisis at the start of our work together.

For some people compulsive caregiving turns into a way of feeling powerful and in control of the world around them. It makes them be the strong one, the hero who is always coping in a crisis, the rock that everybody can lean on when they are in trouble. And while a person may still experience a resonance with feelings of need and terror in others, these feelings are now just this: in others, rather than in themselves. This makes it safe to engage with them and find ways of making them better. Some ignored children who function like this choose to become members of a helping profession, including the profession of psychotherapy.

In these people, there is a spectrum between feeling a strong kinship with sufferers based on their own suffering (the "Wounded Healers") and being completely disconnected from their own suffering to the point of going to great lengths in order to make sure that the suffering is somebody else's. In either case, the ability to effectively help the other will depend on the helper's ability to hold both their own suffering and the other person's in mind, and at the same time to maintain them as separate, so that they can perceive the difference between themselves and those they want to help. It will also depend on the helper's relationship with their own power and how well this has been worked through in their own therapy.

The main difficulty with this coping mechanism is that underneath the compassionate and helpful exterior there is still a core that feels hollow, not seen, not understood, and not loved. This core is probably well shut away and protected. However, many compulsive caregivers know that this core is still there, and they experience the compulsive caregiving as a false self. As a consequence, it may be difficult or impossible for this core of the person to receive the appreciation, love, and gratitude that it needs and that it deserves for its efforts. Instead, positive feedback will likely go to the false self and will therefore make the person feel more fragmented. This can contribute substantially to the tendency of compulsive caregivers to ward off positive feedback.

Compulsive caregivers with this core very strongly walled off are at risk of burning out. It is usually possible to spot the early warning signs of giving from a place that does not have much to give and feeling that other people's needs become demands rather than opportunities to express love. If this state of affairs continues for too long, it can become dangerous and presage burnout.

Some compulsive caregivers know that underneath they are unhappy and unloved and profoundly lonely people. For these, life is painful, and it may take a lot of hard work to reverse the dynamic enough so that they can take in some good. Others identify with the caregiver role to the extent that they forget the unhappiness underneath and may only wonder vaguely why it is so vitally important for them to be useful in the world.

On the whole, compulsive caregiving is an extremely successful coping mechanism, as well as a socially necessary and laudable one. This contributes to making it very difficult to change in psychotherapy— there often is not enough motivation to change and too much gain in maintaining it. After all, it is gratifying to be told forever that you should look after yourself more and not always put others first. Add to that the inclination of the world around compulsive caregivers to want them to continue doing what they do and often to respond in seriously unpleasant ways when they start to change! So it seems important to me to remember that this coping mechanism is bought at a terrible price, that underneath it is a small person who has been ignored and perhaps forgotten, who does not deserve that fate.

CHAPTER 2

Possible Scenarios
of Emotional Neglect

At this point I feel it is necessary to say something about what may have happened in the lives of ignored children. This is both to clarify what I mean by saying somebody has been emotionally neglected, to make some statements about the role of caregivers—especially parents—in people's lives, and to suggest ways of thinking about that role.

I use the terms *emotionally neglected* and *ignored* more or less interchangeably, because I think being ignored is essentially the experience of being emotionally neglected. It means having caregivers who are not tuned in to the emotional well-being of a child, who don't see signs of distress (or choose to ignore them), and who don't reliably respond to a child's appeal for help, comfort, or empathy. They may act like this out of ignorance, or out of their own psychological problems, or because they are not physically present. It includes caregivers who don't wonder whether the child is well but assume that they are okay—or don't want to know. Of necessity it includes caregivers who are often absent, either physically not there or psychologically not present, in the sense of being preoccupied with something else or extremely withdrawn.

Among caregivers whose behavior can give rise to emotionally neglected children, I don't include caregivers who have educational goals that are different from the emotional well-being of their child (such as a good education, making a good marriage, surviving conditions of hardship) but who within their own belief system can be called caring. However, I am aware that there may be cases in which a caregiver's preoccupation with their main educational aim may become all-consuming to the degree that their parenting does deserve the term emotional neglect. For example, a caregiver who is totally focused on raising a child to be a film star from an early age, and who ignores the child's needs in this preoccupation, may well be emotionally neglectful.

The healthy opposite of neglect is attention, or an experience of being seen, cared about, and held in mind. There is also an unhealthy opposite, namely invasion, and most children experience being invaded as a form of more or less subtle abuse. Quite a lot of research has been done into how much attention children need. As a result of this, we can say that there is a healthy medium between too much and too little attention, and thus we can speak of *healthy neglect* that a child can experience—neglect that stretches and grows the child's ability to look after their own needs, while still knowing that in an emergency help is available. This kind of experience then provides a child with space to just be by themself (Beebe & Lachmann, 2002) and makes them feel that they are not invaded or overly controlled by their caregivers. What is healthy neglect will depend on the individual child as well as the quality of the caregivers' attention and other, more external, circumstances. The needs of a child for attention will also not always be the same, but there will be times when a child needs more attention; adequate caregiving will mean that this is available.

I am aware that all notions of what degree of neglect of children is acceptable or healthy are also very culturally constructed and have changed dramatically in the course of the last 50 to 100 years. During that time, there has undoubtedly been a shift, at least in Western society, from a concern with the material well-being of children (including their education and general provision for a successful life) to a concern with their happiness and self-actualization. I don't think this means that emotional neglect was the norm 50 or 100 years ago—I believe that children would have experienced care from their caregivers even if that care didn't focus on their emotional well-being. Equally in cultures in which nowadays parents may have perfectly good reasons for not putting the emotional well-being of their children in the center of family life, this does not of itself constitute emotional neglect.

Those for whom the term emotionally neglected is appropriate have missed a sense of concern, of internal participation, of being seen as separate human beings from their caregivers that is more a measure of the quality of the contact with their caregivers than its quantity. It is this subjective experience of feeling ignored, unloved, taken for granted, merely tolerated, or downright not wanted that I believe leads to the presentation of an ignored child that this book is about. It is very much my experience that this subjective experience may well be present in a situation in which the caregiver is convinced they are the most loving parent in the world. People's experiences of relationships vary so widely that the caregiver's good and loving intentions are simply no guarantee that a child will feel cared for.

I want to emphasize the point that in my experience most caregivers will say that they have the best possible intentions. They may on occasion act contrary to these, for instance when they are angry, stressed, or frightened. They may or may not be aware of such lapses, and they may be busy telling themselves a story about their behavior that preserves their own good opinion of themselves. Or they may just have done the best they could in difficult circumstances. I want to respect their point of view. It is not my intention to provide ammunition for those who are out to attack or blame their caregivers. On the other hand, it is also not my intention to go along with any stories that there is nothing wrong and a person had a perfect childhood—when they are patently suffering from emotional neglect. I have never yet met anybody who was willfully or randomly anxious or depressed; there are always reasons, and the way a person is generally represents the result of their best efforts.

This is relevant for the therapy of adults who were ignored children. Most adults who were ignored children have very insecure attachments to their caregivers, and this manifests in their tendency to protect them. It is very common for ignored children to say that they can't bear to think poorly of their parents. However, these ignored children most assuredly need to separate from their caregivers, and in this process, they need to find their own narrative of their childhood, rather than to buy into their caregivers'. Sometimes it is helpful in this process to put some blame on the caregivers and get angry with them. Sometimes it is more helpful to support clients' understanding that to explore their own subjective experience of their childhood does not mean we want to blame and vilify their parents. In saying this, I am also aware that for many people, it is difficult to hold in mind the possibility that both parents and child may have had good intentions and done their best, and the outcome may still be enormous suffering for the child.

Like most psychotherapy clients, clients who were ignored children often grapple with the issue of whether to have a conversation with their caregivers about the adverse childhood experiences they have had—assuming their caregivers are still around. There needs to be a weighing up of the benefits of creating a better here-and-now relationship between adults and their caregivers through bringing their version of events into the contact, versus protecting the client's own narrative and possibly the caregivers' narrative of their own lives as well. In an ideal world, we hope that the client can have a conversation with their caregiver that expresses some of their experience and feelings about it, without attacking or blaming the caregiver, for the sake of the truth in what is likely to be a lifelong relationship.

There can be many reasons why a child does not have an appropriate place in their parents' lives. Parents may be absent because of external circumstances, or they may be preoccupied with other things including their marriage or other relationships, their health, work-related problems, financial issues, siblings who need a lot of attention for whatever reason, other relatives such as elderly parents who need a lot of care, and so on—ordinary life kinds of issues, in fact. For periods of time this is normal and probably not a bad thing. Sometimes parents just need to be able to rely on a child being okay without constant care and attention, and for the child it is an opportunity to be a little more independent and autonomous than usual. Damage can be assumed to become more likely when the situation goes on for a long time or is very severe and where there are no other caregivers available at all. It is probably only in an ideal world that those who plan to have children would take into consideration the stability of their life circumstances and the availability of the necessary resources for providing their children with the consistent care and attention they need.

There are also cases in which the caregivers are preoccupied with a codependent or abusive relationship, or with substances like alcohol or drugs, or a serious mental illness such as depression or OCD. In these cases, it is more obvious to all concerned that the children just don't get the attention that they need and will suffer as a consequence. For many ignored children this makes it easier to understand why they are suffering.

The situation is worse when both parents are preoccupied, so that there isn't anyone available to go to when the child really needs something. The consequences for later life are also more deleterious when the parental preoccupation happens early in the child's life rather than later. Infants and babies are far more dependent on reliable good contact, and disruptions will have much more serious effects on them than on older children. This is true despite the fact that children will not, of course, remember such disruptions in later life—but the memories will be laid down in implicit form and affect the person well into adulthood.

There are probably many parents who don't particularly enjoy infants and babies but enjoy older children much more, and children of such parents may or may not feel in later life that they were ignored, depending on the severity of the lack of early bonding. It seems to make a difference not only at what age a child was neglected—the younger the child was, the more devastating the consequences tend to be—but also how long it lasted, and whether it ever changed or just continued until the child was grown up (see also Straus & Kantor, 2005).

Again, I do not believe it necessary for every emotionally neglected child to find somebody to blame. There is a therapeutic use for blaming an outside agent when a client is very trapped in self-blaming. In these cases, putting blame on a person or circumstance outside the client is a helpful stage in a process of separation. On the whole, I am using subjective experience to define emotional neglect because I want to avoid blame. Psychotherapy is not usually in a position to determine who is responsible or to blame for a situation, but is concerned with the viewpoint of the client, knowing full well that others may have a different experience of the same events. My life has taught me that things can go very wrong, and people can get very badly hurt, without anybody having a malicious intention toward another.

I also don't think it is helpful to blame parents for being absent, depressed, or preoccupied. I understand, and feel it is important to validate, that the sons and daughters of these parents are angry because they have suffered. I also understand that their parents may not be open to owning their own shortcomings, and indeed their perceived shortcomings may not consist of anything more than ignorance and lack of skill. While I can see the use of blame as a temporary measure in a psychotherapeutic process, I also feel that from the viewpoint of what constitutes a good life in a good world, blaming others is extremely problematic and potentially destructive. It therefore seems to me more helpful for the righteous anger of clients who were ignored children to be expressed elsewhere—perhaps in therapy.

What I can recommend to ignored children is that they focus on themselves, on their own narrative. It is often part of being emotionally neglected—and therefore feeling the need to preserve the tenuous relationships they have—that clients who were ignored children are too understanding of the caregivers' point of view, most likely out of loyalty to their caregivers. This makes the therapy more difficult, and there needs to be a shift from taking the (often "reasonable") viewpoint of the caregiver to taking the viewpoint of the neglected child. I am passionate about affirming the subjective experience that each of my clients has had and about questioning how much it is contaminated with other people's narratives, especially when these other people have an agenda. It is important for clients to be loyal to themselves in order to have a good therapy outcome, far more important than to be able to get their caregivers to admit fault or make restitution. Loyalty toward themselves, even a passion for caring for themselves, is a quality that I aim to grow in all my clients. Once this has been established, it is usually also easier for appropriate gratitude toward our caregivers to be felt and expressed.

In the following, I will describe in a bit more detail the possible scenarios that we may find in clients with a history of emotional neglect.

Absent Caregivers

The simplest possibility for a scenario that leads to emotional neglect is an absent caregiver. This may include absences of mothers because of physical illness including perinatal medical complications; the death of the mother; or the removal of an infant from the mother when the infant is to be fostered or adopted. It may also include infants who had to be isolated from the rest of the world, such as premature infants who needed to be in an incubator, although nowadays nursing staff mostly do their utmost to provide adequate physical and emotional contact for these infants (World Health Organization, 2013). In people older than about 50 the possibility still needs to be considered that they may have been abandoned for some time as infants or young children if they were born prematurely or with a serious medical condition. In all these cases there may have been a period of days, weeks, or even months when the infant did not have an appropriate attachment figure available, and this can impact the infant very greatly and have lifelong consequences.

Olivia was given up for adoption by her mother just after birth. She has seen her adoption file and knows that she remained in hospital for some weeks until a foster family was found for her. She then stayed with this foster family until she was about 6 months old and was moved to the family that later adopted her. We can see from this that her early attachment history is a severely disrupted one—she can only ever had time to form a very tenuous attachment until each caregiver disappeared and she had to start with a new one. By the time she was adopted, she would have formed an internal working model of the world as an unreliable and unsafe place where her own welcome was by no means assured. Tragically, her adopted parents failed to understand this and interpreted her fear and insecurity as a lack of gratitude. "So I learned very early that my parents needed me to be grateful above all, and that I needed to express my gratitude to them if I wanted to be accepted. Because of this, gratitude became a terrible duty so that I ended up hating the very word. Of course, it would have been unimaginably worse if I had ever let anybody see this."

Many adults who were adopted as babies have wounds that go back to a sense of doubtful welcome in the world. How much they struggle with life tends to depend on whether there was a period of time between being taken from their genetic parents and being adopted, and how long this period was, as well as whether their experience at the hands of either set of parents was in itself traumatic.

One of the very serious tragedies in a child's life is the death of a parent at an early age, especially if that parent was the main caregiver. Research that has been available since the 1950s and 1960s shows clearly the connection between depression and early loss of a caregiver and the importance of loving care and attention from alternative care-givers in order to mitigate the damage done by the bereavement (Emde, Polak, & Spitz, 1965; Robertson & Robertson, 1989; Spitz, 1965). In addition to suffering from the loss, these children may consciously or unconsciously blame themselves for the death of the parent. Often enough they will be blamed by other family members; it is not uncommon that when a woman dies in childbirth, the rest of the family will then blame the child for this in such a way that the child grows up with a clear message of being bad or dangerous.

Norman lost his mother when he was only 3 years old, so he was really too young to understand what was happening. This makes his suffering particularly poignant as it is devoid of a narrative; there

43

is just a sense of dull and joyless enduring. He vaguely remembers that in the time after his mother's death, he was handed around the extended family who took turns to look after him for a few weeks at a time. Every time he had settled in with a caregiver he was passed on to the next person. He depicts this as a very bleak time. "I don't think I was very interested in my caregivers, and they certainly weren't interested in me. I just wanted my mother back, or at least to be with my father. But that didn't happen, and the various aunts just kept telling me that my father didn't have time for me. So I gave up and just tried to survive stoically. But I think my relatives thought I was being sullen and bad-tempered, and I remember people telling me to cheer up and giving me a hard time for being such a sullen child. I think I have never really come out of this depression: it has become my home," he says.

Depressed Caregivers

Postpartum depression is a common occurrence. A substantial proportion of all women experience depressed feelings for a few days immediately after giving birth—the so-called baby blues. Usually this passes very quickly and does not interfere with normal bonding between the mother and her baby, but in a proportion of women the state persists for weeks or months and is also more serious (Murray, 1992; Murray & Cooper, 1996). When that happens, we can assume that there will be consequences for the baby that may last well into adulthood.

Many people believe that such postnatal depression is caused by the hormonal changes that accompany the birth of a child. Others have argued against this (D. Rowe, personal communication, 2008). However that may be, it is clear from research that many psychological factors contribute heavily, such as a previous history of depression; lack of emotional support for the woman, including the support from her partner and from her own mother; and how difficult or even traumatic the experience of the birth itself has been (Field et al., 2008; Milgrom et al., 2008; Reynolds, 1997).

When a new mother is seriously depressed, the result for the baby is that they have a mother who is unresponsive, preoccupied, and withdrawn, and may have periods of bad temper (Cori, 2017). As the baby is heavily dependent on having a responsive caregiver for their emotional and physical well-being, this is a terrible situation and will result in deficits in the psychological makeup of the baby. Not only will the feeling of an initial welcome to the world, an initial joy in a caregiver's eyes and a first enveloping and warming love be missing, but also there will be an absence of mirroring, of little bits of communication, and of attuned responses to the baby's experience. Ed Tronick has created the Still Face experiment that demonstrates just how distressing it is for a small person if their caregiver does not respond (Cohn & Tronick, 1983; Weinberg et al., 2008). Some video footage of such experiments is available on the internet and makes for very harrowing viewing, especially for viewers who may have had depressed mothers (Tronick, 2009). The Still Face experiment lasts only for a few seconds at a time, but that is long enough for the baby's fragile ego defenses to crumble very substantially, down to the point where motor coordination is partly lost; it is hard to imagine the consequences if the situation went on and on for weeks or months. We do know that the development of the baby's brain can be seriously impaired by such an experience.

Mortimer asks his parents one day about the circumstances of his own birth. His mother immediately says, "Oh, it was terrible. I had thought it would not be a big deal to have a baby, but the birth was incredibly long and painful, so I swore to myself afterwards

I'd never have another baby. And it took me months to recover—both physically because I had such large and painful scars, and also emotionally because I was so disappointed with myself for finding it all so difficult. The lack of sleep really got to me, and your father didn't help much, and for about a year I just seemed to get more and more depressed. It was only after your first birthday that things started to improve a little, but really, looking back, I think I was depressed for years." Mortimer is startled, because she has never told him this. It throws him into an orgy of guilty feelings, even though he knows rationally that he cannot be blamed for his mother's difficulties. He is so identified with her that he cannot help but feel he has somehow injured his mother just by being born. It takes a long time in his therapy to fill in his own experience as a baby, which would have been a very miserable and difficult one. For me the narrative also makes more sense of the observation that he is prepared to do absolutely anything if it makes his mother happy.

I find that clients who have had depressed mothers typically share certain characteristics. They have a history of being remarkably compliant children who were anxious underneath the compliant mask. Moreover, they often live in a kind of emotional fog where feelings are not very clear in nature and are difficult to access. This can be seen as the direct consequence of the lack of early mirroring. How badly they suffer will depend on how well or poorly supported their mothers were. If there were other caregivers who cared for the baby during the mother's depressed phase, the damage will be less. If a person has many experiences of being left in the care of a very depressed parent, they will have spent part of their childhood in a kind of prison where there was too much stillness, not enough contact, not enough play, and too much time having to just wait and be good.

Preoccupied Caregivers

Some caregivers are so preoccupied with themselves and their own needs that they neglect the needs of the children in their care. In this category fall all the parents who have difficulties taking on the responsibility of being a parent and who will only at times behave according to this role (Gibson, 2015). Here we also find mothers who are still children themselves or who are so needy that they feel themselves to be in competition with their baby for care and attention and may end up feeling envious of anything they give their baby. There are also parents who see their children as an extension of themselves rather than as separate human beings. There are those who treat their children as fashion accessories or as the idealized version of themselves that they would have liked to be. There are all the parents who use their children in order to feel loved by somebody (because everybody knows that children love you unconditionally and always will) and in order to get the parenting that they themselves have not had. We can see from this that such parents may well have been ignored children themselves who pass the problems on to the next generation.

All these are emotionally unavailable caregivers, caregivers who lack the consistent ability to engage with the children in their care, see them as separate people, feel an interest in who they are and how they are, and set a high priority on their emotional well-being. The children in their care are very likely to be ignored and emotionally neglected.

They will most likely also be heavily parentified and may become compulsive caregivers. They will be the people who spend their lives trying to make their parents happy and possibly trying to be something they are not. They may also spend their childhood trying to pacify, placate, or control their parents. They often have a hard time working out later what their problem is, because they may not realize that their caregivers were preoccupied to the point of neglecting them. It is also possible that their caregivers will feel attacked and shamed and will fight back if they are told there is something wrong with their caregiving!

Olivia and I work at length on the issues connected to her being given up for adoption by her genetic mother. Eventually we start to examine her adopted parents a little more closely and she begins to appreciate the difficulties that she experienced living with them. It becomes clear that she often got told off for no very good reason and at these times invariably felt herself to be a bad person. When we start to unpack this kind of experience, she tells me that thinking she was bad enabled her to preserve the good feelings she had toward her adopted mother. We are both struck with how her mother's relentless need for Olivia's gratitude represents a powerful self-idealization that left no option to her child than to become the "bad" one and take the blame and the shame for anything that went wrong. Olivia starts to feel more compassion for her younger self as she realizes that this was sometimes the only way she could love her mother.

I think that in this category we also find the children with the greatest difficulties separating from their caregivers. This is because their caregivers are quite likely to have behaved in an inconsistent way, sometimes caring for their children and sometimes ignoring them, and there will have been no discernible pattern to this inconsistency. Biological experiments have long established that an inconsistent response creates the greatest difficulty in letting go of anything good, and this applies to animals as well as to humans (Crum, Brown, & Bitterman, 1951; Dwairy, 2008; Pittenger, 2002). Children of parents whose availability is inconsistent will spend an inordinate amount of time and energy trying to figure out the pattern or rule. This is a trait that can survive into adulthood and create much misery among those who were ignored children. Another result of inconsistent caregiver availability may well be that the child, and later the adult, has memories of good care that they have received. It may be difficult to discern just how inconsistent this care was. This will make it that much harder to understand the symptoms of emotional neglect for these clients. They may well feel great shame for being as they are, given that they do have good memories.

I also include under this heading the caregivers who were preoccupied for different reasons, such as being addicted to a substance; or being preoccupied with a difficult, possibly abusive relationship with a partner; or being preoccupied with their own physical or mental health or that of a spouse, parent, or another child. The result of these preoccupations will also be parentified children who spend their lives trying to heal their parents' wounds and making them better. They will have the advantage of a narrative for their fate and thus fewer difficulties understanding how they have come to be as they are. In addition, the ignored children in this category may have a degree of overlap with other presentations.

In the course of therapy, Pearl grows very conscious of how little she felt seen as a child. "My mother probably couldn't really forgive me for being the wrong gender, and it must have meant that she was not interested in me. And on top of that, there were these endless hours of her complaining about my father to me, going on and on about him and his many shortcomings. When I think of my childhood, it's hard to remember any other topic of conversation with my mother. She seemed completely eaten up by her unhappiness about my father. I remember feeling that she wanted me to look after her and make it all better. And I so desperately wanted to make her happy, but it hardly ever worked."

Overlap with Other Presentations

It is quite difficult to find clients who have a history of emotional neglect and only that. Mostly we will find that ignored children also had traumatic experiences, perhaps because they were left to cope with things from which other children would be protected. Many ignored children were also neglected physically, be it because of extreme poverty of the family or because their caregivers also ignored their physical needs (Grassi-Oliveira & Stein, 2008; Nikulina & Widom, 2014). In fact, we can probably make the opposite assumption: if somebody has been neglected physically as a child, we can assume that they have also been neglected emotionally.

Often we find in clinical practice that emotional neglect overlaps with abuse of some kind: emotional, physical, or sexual. This makes sense when we remember that emotionally neglected children get ignored, and so their caregivers are unlikely to hold their safety and well-being in mind as a first priority. Sadly, there are also parents whose emotional unavailability alternates with emotional cruelty or abusive behavior. It can also be argued that just as neglect is a form of abuse, so abuse is a form of neglect: a breakdown of empathy and a lack of attention to the needs of the child are certainly common to both (Brown, 2014; Hopper et al., 2018; Norman et al., 2012; Taillieu et al., 2016; Widom, 1999).

In many cases we can identify early trauma or early loss without necessarily finding evidence of emotional neglect, but often the two will go together. For instance, if a parent has died in early childhood, the surviving parent may not have coped well with caring for the child and may subsequently have ignored them.

To conclude, the presentation of being ignored often doesn't come in the pure form that I am describing here but mixed up with other presentations. I want to emphasize that working with the more traumatic events in a person's life should not distract us entirely from looking at emotional neglect—otherwise we are caught in an enactment where we repeat the emotional neglect of our clients. The example of Olivia's story above illustrates the importance of addressing emotional neglect separately and at length.

Finally, I want to make the point that the deleterious effects of abuse are greatly enhanced by neglect and vice versa. Both are factors that will elevate the baseline of stress in the child's body and mind, and therefore the resulting stress will be the consequence of both. Moreover, as emotional neglect undermines a person's resourcefulness and resilience, any traumatic incidents will happen to a person who is highly vulnerable in the first place, and therefore the impact of further stress is likely to be potentiated. There is therefore a strong case for saying that if psychotherapy is able to address both abuse and neglect in a person's history, the therapy will therefore be that much more effective and most probably also faster.

CHAPTER 3

Psychotherapeutic Theories About Ignored Children

In this chapter I will start to look at how we can fit our understanding of ignored children into a theoretical framework, which is necessary if we are to formulate therapeutic strategies.

I want to begin by stating my basic philosophical stance in psychotherapy, in the hope that this will help readers understand how I am choosing to represent theories in this section and how I integrate them into an overarching system. My *model of mind* is essentially a developmental one. I believe that there is such a thing as a developmental urge, a motive force that is trying to develop as we progress in life. This force seems to me to be related to our vitality and our creativity, emerging as an expression of life in the whole organism. It aims to develop a broader range of resources and a greater degree of complexity in the mind and will thus over time create more adaptive ways of living.

Development from birth happens in stages, and early in each stage, a new development is particularly vulnerable and can be discouraged. When this happens, it will collapse and be given up. If development is discouraged later in the same developmental stage, it will be repressed but persist in a repressed form, to be reactivated if the repression is lifted. The two possibilities are different: in the first case, the developmental gain does not happen at all, whereas in the second case, the developmental gain is still there albeit in a hidden form. In the physical body, the first case will lead to a body part lacking tone and vitality and feeling cold and empty, whereas the second part will lead to a part that holds too much tone and vitality and feels hot and full. The psychological counterparts will have similar qualities that can be experienced by the person themself and also in interpersonal contact by others. Developmental deficits such as we find as a result of emotional neglect are an example of the first case; neurotic conflicts are an example of the second case.

There is also the possibility that previously attained developmental steps are relinquished as a result of very severe trauma and will then present as if they had never happened (M. Holm Brantbjerg, personal communication, 2019).

In individual instances, both in the context of normal development and of trauma, giving up or repressing may not be a simple binary choice; rather there may be a spectrum across which an individual will attempt to salvage aspects of a developmental gain while giving up others. However, one of the two usually dominates, so that overall a personality trait can be experienced as either given up or repressed.

Development happens in many stages, and things can go well or less well at any point. When things have gone badly at an early stage, later stages will be affected but will probably happen anyway, albeit in a modified form that may lack resilience or be distorted in some fashion Some events have more deleterious effects than others. Being shamed appears to be one of the more harmful events in terms of its effect on the later development of the person. This may be because in order to develop at all, a person needs a degree of confidence in their own ability to do so, and overwhelming shame seems to inhibit this confidence. We can almost think of shame as inhibiting developmental impulses at their root.

My understanding of ignored children is consistent with this model of mind. For details, I draw much of my understanding from two main bodies of theory: one is attachment theory, and the other is body psychotherapy. Attachment theory has contributed the understanding of insecure attachment and what the consequences are in later life. Body psychotherapy has contributed an emphasis on self-regulation, which is difficult for ignored children. It has also contributed the more descriptive concepts of the schizoid and the oral characters, which represent sets of habitual coping strategies (ego defenses) typically adopted by people with early childhood trauma. There is a substantial amount of overlap between these different categories, but they were developed in different contexts, so it seems worthwhile exploring both for their therapeutic usefulness with ignored children. Perhaps most important, branches of body psychotherapy have developed an understanding of clients who mostly suffer from developmental deficits.

This chapter focuses on theoretical understanding and will therefore emphasize the helpfulness of different approaches for deepening our understanding of ignored children's experience. It will not focus on specific therapeutically fruitful interventions. Such therapeutic interventions can be found in Chapter 6. Having said that, we need to bear in mind that understanding and the resulting empathy and compassion are very powerful therapeutic interventions in their own right and may constitute much of what some ignored children need in order to heal. Moreover, theories help therapists to contain much distress and be more present with their clients, which also adds to the success of good psychotherapy.

Attachment Theory and Avoidant Attachment Style

Few theoretical concepts have changed the world of psychotherapy as dramatically as John Bowlby's attachment theory (Bowlby, 1951, 1969,

1973). Initially, attachment theory was intended as a purely descriptive and phenomenological approach to looking at the kinds of bonds that small children form with their caregivers. It was soon recognized that people could be categorized according to their attachment style and that this often remained constant throughout life (Ainsworth et al., 1978; Main, 1985).

Attachment styles fall into four categories: a secure attachment style and three styles of insecure attachment. Insecure attachment is divided into ambivalent (also called resistant or, in adults, preoccupied), avoidant (in adults called dismissive), and disorganized (see for example, Wallin, 2007).

Attachment theory thus distinguishes among the following four possibilities:

1. If a baby experiences their caregiver as available for contact reliably and in a way that leaves the baby feeling seen and adequately attended to, the attachment will be secure. This baby will be able to move in and out of contact with the caregiver relatively easily and without being unbearably distressed. A secure attachment will be a good basis for a gradual process of separation.

2. If the baby experiences the caregiver as insufficiently available for contact but unavailable in such a way that there seems to be hope for the attachment to get better, the baby keeps trying to improve the situation and ends up in an ambivalent attachment. This attachment style is called ambivalent because the sustained effort to be sufficiently attached also leaves considerable negativity in the baby, which can get expressed in angry pushing away, particularly when the caregiver returns from an absence.

3. If on the other hand the baby experiences the caregiver as largely unavailable with little or no hope of better availability, the baby will

start to avoid attempts to make contact in order to protect themself from the pain of the rejection. This results in an avoidant attachment style in which the baby appears to have lost interest in the caregiver.

4. Finally, in situations in which the same caregiver is sometimes experienced as caring and loving and sometimes as frightening, attacking, or abusive, the baby's attachment ends up completely disorganized and the baby will go into life with a considerable load of trauma and usually an inability to know what constitutes good contact.

When looking more closely at how attachment bonds are formed, researchers have found that they arise out of close physical contact and involve processes of mirroring and resonance. It has been shown that the nonsensical-seeming little proto-conversations that most people will spontaneously engage in when in contact with a baby are in fact the stuff of attachment (Schore, 1994; Stern, 1991; Trevarthen, 1993; Wallin, 2007). These little sequences typically consist of a beginning (making contact), a middle (interacting) and an ending (withdrawing from the contact). In such interactions babies learn the flavor of human communication and the shape of contact and experience predictability and reliability of good care. In the absence of words, these interactions are carried out through eye contact, facial expression, touch, and gestures. Such proto-conversations have been shown to be highly musical and thus have internal rules and predictability (Gratier & Trevarthen, 2008). They satisfy the sense that seems innate in all of us of *story*, of processes that happen in an orderly fashion from beginning to end. They are the kinds of interactions that create meaning in a world that might otherwise be confusing and bewildering. In these interactions, the baby gets an opportunity to have their feelings mirrored by the caregiver, who can contribute the experience of a grown-up person and carry a feeling through to a resolution, making it safe and manageable for the baby. Over time the baby will internalize the way such episodes run their course, and this will become the internal map of the world that the baby has for the future, perhaps for the rest of their life.

This process is called affect regulation and has been described at length (Gerhardt, 2004; Hart, 2008; Schore, 1994). It forms not only our internal map for relationships with other humans that will be with us all our lives, but also the core of our own sense of self: the way we handle life and its vicissitudes. Experiences of challenge, struggle, failure, or achievement are rooted in these early interactions. Our basic expectations of the world as helpful, indifferent, or hostile arise directly from them. Our ability to cope with difficulties will critically depend on this, leading to a sense of self as more or less effective in the world and a life that is going to be more or less stressful.

If we think of a baby who tries to make contact with the caregiver and meets with a caregiver who has no time, no interest, or no inclination to engage, we can imagine what happens: the baby learns that trying to make contact leads to rejection and abandonment and the terrible pain and fear associated with this. The baby learns that the world is not interested and may be hostile; people will not help or make anything better; and the baby needs to look after themself in order to survive. The baby is also likely to conclude that they are not desirable, not particularly welcome, and not effective at making good contact. Expressing feelings, especially feelings of anger or protest, may well elicit retaliation from the caregivers. It thus becomes something to be avoided. The baby cannot develop a belief that it is in any way helpful to communicate internal experience to others and instead learns to avoid contact. Avoidantly attached babies are usually very compliant and turn into compliant, "good" children. Tragically, this may encourage their caregivers to ignore them further because they don't appear to need anything and always present a facade of being fine to the world. In many ignored children, there is no experience that might suggest that the world has any help or support to offer—instead they experience themselves as utterly powerless to affect their environment or elicit cooperation from another human. Some ignored children may be aware that their own behavior of avoiding reaching out for help or support contributes to their plight. Chances are that to change this will create too much anxiety for them to handle, so they will feel either aggrieved or ashamed of themselves but unable to change the situation. The typical train of thought will be, "I can't get what I want but if I protest or ask for anything, my caregivers will be angry and deny me what I need, anyway. So my only, albeit slim, chance is to be good and hope that one day somebody will recognize this and reward me."

This kind of history is very close to what I think Pearl must have experienced. She certainly spent her childhood being very compliant in the hope of getting some crumbs of affection from a mother who barely had time for her. Now, as an adult, it is one of her beliefs that other people don't cooperate and will not help—she has to do everything she wants done. Mostly she is capable of doing that, and this capability gives her a good feeling of competence and power, but it is severely unbalanced because receiving support, help, or care are really unknown experiences for her. This kind of unbalanced lifestyle is unsustainable. It may be maintained while doing everything for herself is met with tolerance or affirmation by her environment; but when it is met with negativity, as is happening for Pearl currently, she is at a very high risk of burning out.

The term *avoidantly attached* is often understood to mean that a person does not feel much distress at separation or loss. This can be misleading in clinical practice. While we do encounter avoidantly attached clients who find separations easy and are comfortable in their own company, we also find those who spend their lives desperately clinging to very tenuous early attachment relationships. Indeed, this clinging to a few desperately insecure attachments is often found in the same people who in most relationships can easily separate. It may manifest as exaggerated loyalty to, as strong identification with, or as a determined idealization of their attachment figures. Nearly always it will manifest in tremendous difficulties separating from attachment figures. We may feel that the person is hanging on to something well beyond the time when it would be much more sensible to give up and go elsewhere. I usually get the image of somebody who has just had a glimpse or two of what it would be like to be loved and cared for and safe and who then spends their life desperately hoping for the return of this state of bliss that may remain forever beyond their reach. Therefore, my sense of ignored children is that they are often on an edge between being avoidantly and ambivalently attached, and their need to hold on to what feels like everything they have got in the world is incredibly powerful.

My example of this type of attachment is Norman. The strength of his holding on to attachment figures is very clear in the therapeutic relationship with me. Presumably the original attachment figure to whom he so desperately clings is his mother, who died when he was only 3 years old. He manifestly feels the powerful loyalty to his mother that I would expect. Now attachment theory teaches us that attachments are most likely difficult to let go of when they have not been secure—as if the child has not had enough of the relationship. I therefore have a suspicion that Norman's attachment to his mother was an insecure one in the first place: at the very least her long illness would have disrupted the bond between them, and it seems likely that the bond was never a very robust one. This is relevant for the therapy because I am expecting to find an insecure pattern in Norman's attachment to me, and I have to keep in mind that there may not be a blueprint for a more secure attachment relationship. I may therefore have to start from a long way down with building some relational security.

I want to emphasize the image that avoidantly attached people who present for therapy may have glimpsed moments of secure attachment. A helpful concept is that we separate from anything good when we have had enough of it, and if we only ever catch glimpses of a good thing, we can never get enough. Having enough of anything includes spending time immersing ourselves and really savoring and having it, so that we can make it our own. Then, when the process of internalizing and assimilating has run its course, we lose interest entirely naturally and can easily let go.

Attachment theory has contributed an understanding of parentification as a reversal of an attachment relationship, in which the caregiver uses a baby or small child to meet their own attachment needs. It is easy to see that this can result in a compulsive caregiver personality, if the child's attempt to parent the parents is at least partly successful and leads to more safety or more acceptance for the child. This is the scenario in which caregiving becomes an extraordinarily adaptive coping mechanism that can continue for the rest of the person's life. Whether the person will ever feel a need to change this or not may depends on how much care the person is able to give to themselves as well as others. If the caregiving is limited to others in a very black-and-white fashion, and the person has a real terror of receiving anything from others, we can expect that change may never happen and they will burn out at some stage.

Finally, there is an attachment theory formulation of shame, in which shame represents a disruption of an attachment bond that leaves the child exposed and quite possibly extremely unsafe (Kaufmann, 1980). This way of thinking focuses on the experience of shame and of what happens once a person has been shamed (Schore, 1994). The feeling of being exposed, both in the sense of being out of the protective circle of parental care and of being laid open to intrusion and possible violation, is an important aspect of the shame that many ignored children experience. It is as though, because of their very insecure attachment, they are unable to control how much of themselves they share and frequently end up sharing too much for comfort, leading to an experience of shame.

Attachment theory has been enormously influential in the practice of psychotherapy. This may be due partly to its easy accessibility; but it has certainly also been important that many psychotherapists are able to integrate attachment easily into other psychotherapeutic theories (see for example Fonagy, 2001; Wallin, 2007), so that it now forms something of a meeting ground for psychotherapists from very different backgrounds.

Biodynamic Psychotherapy and Emotional Self-Regulation

I now come to the less well-known area of biodynamic psychology and its emphasis on organismic self-regulation (Boyesen, 1980, 1987; Boyesen & Bergholz, 2003; de Brébisson & Brami, 2018; Southwell, 1988). Biodynamic psychology is a submodality of body psychotherapy and the one with perhaps the strongest emphasis on this concept, even though other body psychotherapy submodalities, and indeed other humanistic psychotherapies, tend to include this in their thinking as well.

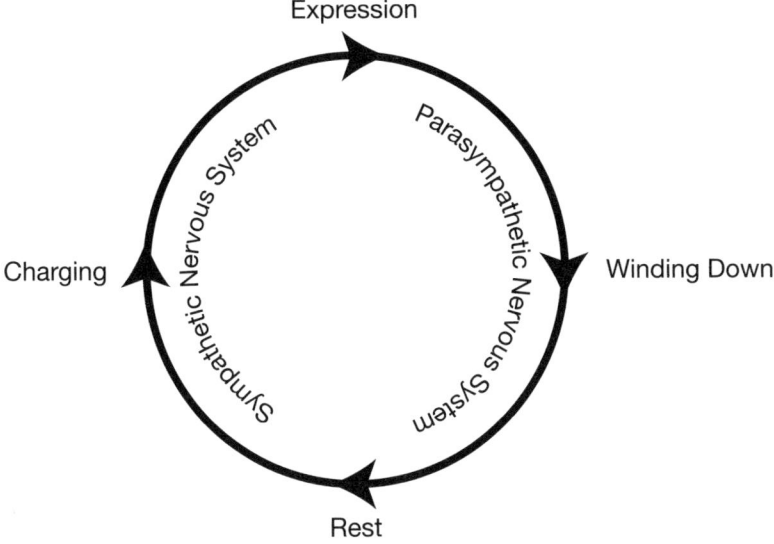

FIGURE 3.1 The Cycle of Self-Regulation as Used in Biodynamic Psychotherapy   Source: Stauffer, K.A. (2010)

Biodynamic psychology was created by Gerda Boyesen, who emphasized the importance of a cycle of self-regulation that she called the vasomotoric cycle (also known as the emotional cycle). The key observation is that the typical sequence of "Charge—Expression—Winding down—Rest" as a basic pattern of life processes is embodied and has a clear physical correlation in the bodily processes governed by the autonomic nervous system (ANS). If we imagine this kind of sequence as a cycle, there is an *upgoing* phase from Rest to Charge to Expression, and a corresponding *downgoing* phase from Expression to Winding down to Rest. The upgoing phase is largely mediated by the sympathetic nervous system, and the physiological processes that get activated include:

- The flow of blood to the skeletal musculature in order to prepare for action;

- Shutting down of all not immediately necessary systems, such as digestion or would healing;
- The pupils of the eyes enlarge and the focal length of the eye lens increases in order to better see what is happening;
- Breath goes into the chest more in order to use the top of the lungs optimally.

Overall these processes produce a shift in the body's energy upwards and outwards. Psychologically, we experience this as activation and a focus on the world around us. The downgoing phase is mediated by the parasympathetic nervous system and includes:

- The redirection of blood flow away from skeletal muscle and toward the skin and the intestines, resulting in a healthier color;
- Activation of the previously shut down processes of digestion and wound healing;
- A decrease in pupil size and focal length of the eye;
- Breath going into the belly more in restorative and relaxing deep breaths.

Overall these processes shift the energy in the body downwards and inwards.

Psychologically, we now experience a letting go and turning our focus inwards. A completed cycle gives us a feeling of achievement, of completion, and of being alive.

We can spot such cycles in every process to do with life, from a simple sequence of breathing in and breathing out, to carrying out a project or task, to how we engage with the world over a lifetime. What is useful is the observation that such cycles rarely run smoothly; everybody tends to have habitual distortions of the cycle that can be observed in every aspect of their life. Thus if we observe how a client manages a therapy session, we may have a very good idea of how they manage challenges, social interactions, and any other areas of their life. There will be the same places where a person always gets stuck and the same places that a person rushes over or takes a shortcut. Observing these patterns gives us a very quick and accurate access to the "how" of a person's self-regulation, and it means that if we can help to smooth the cycles for a client, they will become more resilient and more effective, and they will feel that the therapy is working well.

If we look at these types of cycles from the perspective of the organism engaging in them, we can easily see that the organism is trying to maintain a constant state all the time. In most people's subjective experience, life keeps producing events that throw their inner equilibrium off balance, and then they have to bring it back to their internal home in order to be okay and maintain some internal constancy. Therefore, we can also see these cycles as a way of maintaining a constant internal milieu—something that Antonio Damasio has termed as one of the most important characteristics of a mind (Damasio, 1994, 2000). Biodynamic psychology chooses to focus on the movement as a way of emphasizing the dynamic aliveness in these cycles—but it is good to bear in mind that for ignored children especially, the emphasis on maintaining internal constancy may be the image that they can resonate with more easily (Stauffer, 2009).

It is hard to think of an area of life that is not affected by the quality of self-regulation of which a person is capable. The quality of self-regulation can be experienced both in the level of skill at self-regulating as well as in the degree of dysregulation that the person is able to tolerate without being overly affected. Both of these qualities are, of course, related to each other: the more skills a person has available to self-regulate, the more comfortable they will be to be pushed far away from their home. Both will determine, for example:

- how successfully a person can sustain living in communities including intimate relationships;
- how well a person manages stressful situations in which a lot may be at stake, and therefore how successful they can be;
- how much internal support they have to stand their ground in a competitive and potentially hostile world;
- how much physical resilience a person will have, because an ability to rest and be recharged will be crucial to this;
- how well a person handles physical and psychological trauma, accidents, and illnesses;
- how easily a person can adapt to changes in life circumstances and life stages including adulthood, parenthood, and older age.

Biodynamic psychology differentiates between ways of managing emotions that are more or less healthy. It would for example see shallow breathing (which is essentially a way of reducing the intensity of an emotional experience) as less healthy than an ability to ride the emotion, feel it, and wait for it to subside while breathing fully. Dissociation and going out of one's body would be seen as extreme forms of regulating experience, costing a tremendous price in aliveness and depth of experience. On the other hand, mindful containment of strong emotions would be viewed as a healthy and mature regulatory skill. We can construct hierarchies of self-regulatory skills that closely resemble developmental hierarchies of ego defenses.

Allan Schore has made the very valuable point that this kind of regulation of feelings and experience forms the very stuff of which self is made (Schore, 1994). They form the core of an experience of self as constant over time and as an agent capable of making things better. Those who are unable to self-regulate effectively will be forever dependent on the outside world to help them do this, be that other people, substances (e.g., alcohol, nicotine, or drugs), or specific actions (e.g., exercise or soothing rituals). Either way there will be a level of dependency that will make such a person almost certainly quite emotionally fragile. This unstable state, in which the person feels at the mercy of the world around them, can shift in therapy to a more stable state, in which the person is in contact with an essential solidity and health inside themselves. This shift will profoundly change a person's life and is viewed as an important and highly desirable outcome in biodynamic psychotherapy.

All four of my ignored children have trouble self-regulating adequately. At least on the surface, Mortimer is the most dysregulated and the most difficult to shift into a healthier style of regulation. Because of the apparently total lack of maternal attunement, he has remained extremely anxious and barely in his body for all of his life. From a very early age, he has experienced the barrage of well-meaning suggestions for managing his anxiety as demands that he could not fulfill and that have left him deeply humiliated. Therefore it is now very distressing if I make any kind of suggestion that sounds to him as though I was doing the same thing that his parents and educators did! Once I become aware of this reenactment, I begin to get a handle on the therapy for Mortimer. I invent maneuvers in which I put the emphasis on the two of us doing things together—because I know that he is very good at tuning in to another person. So instead of telling him, for example, to take a deep breath (which he confesses he can't do because he has tried so often and so hard that he has tied himself into impossible knots), I say, "Let's take a breath" and I take a few deep breaths, so that he can just mirror me. I also name how unhelpful many people in his life have been and invite him to let me know how helpful or unhelpful my interventions are. Still, therapy remains slow, and we have to go through many cycles of me making impossible demands and repairing the mistake until he feels secure enough to start self-regulating better in the therapy sessions and in the rest of his life. He also resists this development from a wish to remain attached to me so that I will "do it for him," as well as out of a certain vengefulness that means he feels he is owed an easier life and doesn't want to take all the responsibility for getting better.

The skills for self-regulation people have available form a large part of what psychodynamic therapists call a person's *ego defenses*. To the extent that ego defenses are resources that help people bear strong feelings and protect themselves from being overwhelmed, they are just that—ways of regulating emotional experience. Therefore, all that we know about ego defenses applies to self-regulatory strategies. They can be more or less sophisticated or more or less mature; people add to them as they go through life and as they mature psychologically. When a person is stressed, they lose some of the more sophisticated self-regulatory strategies; they regress. Like ego defenses, these strategies usually involve some kind of compromise between the more spontaneous functions of the personality and more reflective functions, between what the person really wants and what they can get if their anxiety is to be managed at the same time.

Because self-regulatory cycles are embodied and can be tracked in people's bodies (as well as in the quality of contact in the therapeutic relationship), this concept represents a powerful tool for observing how stressed a person is and for teaching clients how to regulate their own stress more effectively. The concept of stress here includes traumatic and post-traumatic stress. It is fairly simple to regard traumatic stress as an extreme state of self-regulation in which body and mind are extremely dysregulated. In psychotherapy, it is of inestimable value to be able to both observe with precision the nonverbal indications that tell us how well our clients are able to assimilate the therapy and also help our clients to do the same outside the therapy room, by fine-tuning their own awareness of how anxious they are at any given moment. For clients who were ignored children and who have usually learned early on to not notice anxious feelings, this fine-tuning can represent a very valuable new resource (Rothschild, 2017). Clients will find it easier to regulate anxiety if their perception of anxiety is more sensitive so that they pick it up before it becomes unmanageably high.

Finally, it is easy to link the biodynamic concepts with the concept of affect regulation that attachment theory uses. The process of affect regulation that can be observed as happening in the relationship of babies and their caregivers leads to an internalization over time, and the result is the emotional self-regulation that we observe in adults in body psychotherapy. We can thus say that self-regulation as we observe it in clients contains its own history and allows us access to it. It is also useful to remember that a person's self-regulation skills may be only as good as their primary caregiver's self-regulation skills, because that is where they mostly come from. More generally we can say that the observable individual nature of a person's self-regulatory habits contains much of the person's history embedded in it.

Working from a biodynamic perspective, psychotherapists would usually start by observing the way a client self-regulates and attempt to get the client also interested in the "how" of their experience. This offers good opportunities to draw out, experience, and underpin the resources that a client already has, an important step in the therapy of ignored children. Then the available self-regulatory skills and resources can be discussed, explored in detail, and built on to grow more in number and complexity. Because self-regulatory cycles can be observed in any part of a person's life, they will be in the therapy room and can be worked on immediately and phenomenologically. A purely phenomenological approach is quite easy to maintain in this context. It has the great advantage of avoiding shame, blame, and judgment and is thus generally easy for clients who were ignored children to engage with.

An added advantage is that biodynamic work tends to improve clients' relationship with their bodies. When clients are in biodynamic psychotherapy for a period of time, they almost invariably report feeling more "in their bodies," being more connected to their biological aliveness, and also more aware of their feelings. I have seen this happen in clients despite body sensation never being mentioned in the therapy. Presumably, learning to co-regulate with me affects how my clients relate to their own bodies implicitly.

One of the strengths of biodynamic work is the ability to slip underneath the client's resistance and contact the deeper and earlier layers of the personality. There is a danger here of the therapy being felt as invasive. However, especially with clients who underneath the need to avoid contact with others have a strong impulse to reach out and find satisfying contact, chances are that the client will feel seen and enjoy the contact. This very enjoyment is healing for ignored children.

Biodynamic psychotherapists tend to be a good match for ignored children. They are generally skilled at picking up nonverbal signals and therefore clients feel understood even when they cannot quite put their experience into words. In addition, most biodynamic psychotherapists are comfortable working with regressed states in an open-ended context. Biodynamic psychotherapists usually use touch and are able to repair to some extent the effects of the touch deprivation that often goes with being ignored. They do this by giving the organism some "good-quality touch" (Carroll, 2002a). The emphasis on body sensation and forms of contact other than verbal communication means that there is generally a good access to preverbal material. It also relieves some ignored children of the pressure to perform by putting internal experiences into language. Biodynamic therapists can hold clients in long and deep processes of regression and reparenting, whereby the client can gradually learn new resources that will support their growth from deep layers of their psyche. Much therapeutic gain may happen without ever using words to describe experience or think about it.

The disadvantage of a biodynamic approach is that for some ignored children, it lacks structure. It may not be helpful to be told to "just let things happen," because that may feel like a demand, and the client may get lost in the confusion of not knowing how to meet this demand. Also, some clients will require an approach that integrates more thinking, speaking, and untangling of issues that get in the way of a completely body-based healing process.

The Schizoid Character Style

The concept of character styles goes back a long way in psychoanalysis. "Character" denotes the set of habitual ego defenses that each of us uses for managing everyday life. In general, these defenses are not experienced as a problem and do not constitute the presenting reason for psychotherapy. In fact, many people are completely oblivious to them and assume that everybody is like this (Reich, 1972).

These defenses are thought to arise from certain events during our early development and thus contain within themselves the history of the developmental period from which they stem. Like all ego defenses, a person's character serves both to ward off unbearable feelings and also to gratify some of the person's needs. Character styles are a very useful map of a person's mind for those therapists who work with the developmental history of their clients. Wilhelm Reich, who wrote extensively on character styles, noticed that to address a person's character defenses usually leads very quickly into the core of the presenting issue.

Reich and, following him, Alexander Lowen, used the term "character structure" to denote the set of ego defenses that is visible in the body structure of a person (Lowen, 1971; Reich, 1972; Totton & Edmondson, 1988). The idea behind this is that, as these defenses arise early on in life, they will shape the development of the skeletal musculature and determine which muscles we use in order to perform certain actions. The habitual use of our muscles in turn can contribute to the shape of the very bones of our bodies, because they may get pulled in characteristic ways as we grow.

Stephen Johnson agrees with this idea but adds the recognition that most people have issues from each major developmental period and therefore a resulting set of defenses, and any of these sets of defenses can be utilized in a given situation. His idea of character is thus more fluid and more complex than Reich's, and he does not limit himself to the character that is laid down in a person's body. I will follow Johnson's terminology because it fits best with my experience (Johnson, 1985, 1994). My clinical practice is also influenced by the synopsis given by Eiden (2002).

I will focus here on the schizoid character style that is thought to arise from events that take place during the perinatal period including the first few months of life. This period includes prenatal events that may have affected the fetus, the birth itself, and much of the attachment period of a baby's life. In the literature, schizoid characters are assumed to have experienced a major trauma during this time; perhaps an attempted termination of the pregnancy or other expression of being unwanted, a very difficult birth, or very early abuse such as being hated by the parents or being given away. Whatever the nature of these events, the baby experiences terror to an extent that cannot be processed, and the only way open to this baby is to go partly out of their body. This may take the form of major dissociation, or a more subtle "not being present," "numbing out," or "getting stuck in the head." Schizoid people are usually very thought-based and typically find it difficult to access feelings—a direct result of not living in their bodies. Their bodies are characterized by deep tensions in the musculature and an unlived-in and rather neglected look. General stiffness and clumsiness may be visible in the physical body and a tendency to look as if the body can only be held together by dint of a supreme effort of willpower. When startled, schizoid people typically freeze; or they may collapse following very little provocation. The body thus presents a look that suggests a tenuous hold on life and not much available vital energy. Therapists may feel that all the vital energy of the person is locked deep inside, perhaps in the bones or joints. A schizoid person has the expectation that they can never be certain of their welcome and that it is not given to them to partake of the fullness of life's abundance. Rather, they may live a carefully delineated existence in the margins, in a little niche that provides them with some safety. Safety is not expected to come from other people, who are experienced as being mostly hard work or downright frightening. In addition to all this terror, schizoid characters are full of rage, which makes the terror worse when felt even a little bit, and which may need addressing at some point.

The typical schizoid character of the literature thus presents a slightly caricatured version of an ignored child. Because the assumed history is a traumatic one, all the expressions of the character style are exaggerated compared with how the kind of client who was an ignored child that I am interested in would present. Many of the traits are there: the preoccupation with safety, the tendency to withdraw from contact when challenged, the tendency not to trust and not to inhabit the body, the defense against needs, the lack of contact with emotions and overreliance on thought. I think of schizoid characters and ignored children as next to each other with a large overlap, but with the distinction that ignored children may not feel hated, just ignored. The result is that ignored children don't have a narrative of how unpleasant their treatment was and typically think that everything was fine and that they are to blame, whereas schizoid characters may have more of an awareness of themselves as victims of some kind. When ignored children finally construct a narrative, it is more commonly one of being unwanted but tolerated; ignored children are more likely to talk about how disgusting and shameful they are on the inside in order to account for being unwanted. We could say that they are less high-functioning than schizoid characters, who see themselves as victims: ignored children may be so identified with their perpetrators that their very victimhood is denied.

Johnson has written one of the most powerful maxims for my own work: remember that a schizoid person has been frightened out of their body and cannot be bullied or frightened back into it (Johnson, 1985). This underpins much of my working style, which is never challenging or confronting. He has also provided us with deep insight into the terrible dilemma where, in order to preserve life, the person needs to not be fully alive.

Olivia has a history of severe perinatal trauma because she was given up for adoption. At one time in her life it was a very palpable reality that she was not welcome. This remains alive in her and colors most of her experience. Her everyday functioning looks fine on the surface but is really quite fragile, and at any moment she is liable to drop into this terrifying world where she has been cast into outer darkness. Her infant mind did what infant minds do: she assumed that this was her own fault. So she has a deep-seated belief that she is bad, disgusting, and hateful. In therapy we develop her thoughts around this and find that keeping the "badness" inside allows her to believe in other people's goodness, and this in turn allows for some hope that she might be redeemed by another. It is this hope that keeps her coming to therapy and also keeps her striving to live a normal life. Sometimes she can almost imagine what it would be like to be told that she is in fact a good person and no longer needs to be ashamed of herself. "But it would probably have to be God himself who tells me this, otherwise I wouldn't believe it," she adds, mindful of her own mistrust of other people.

Her deep sense of not having the right to exist manifests in her body, both as a physical fragility, with many ailments and tendencies to become ill, and also as an impression that she treats her body like a machine: there is no trust that her body can function by itself. At times it almost feels as if Olivia is trying to control its function down to a cellular level. She doesn't feel what her body needs but thinks about what it should need. This fragmentation in itself is not very good for her and creates a lot of stress, stress of which she is no longer even conscious.

The Oral Character Style

Of all the character styles described in the literature, the *oral character* style is the one that most of us find the most difficult to relate to and have the most judgments about. This may be because the central issue is our relationship with our own needs. Words like "needy" and "dependent" have come to acquire very negative and uncomfortable connotations. On the other hand, oral issues are also among the most common in ordinary people as well as in clients who present for psychotherapy. We all have needs and all have to come to terms with our feelings about them and learn to manage them. There are no ideal or permanent solutions; in different periods of our lives we have to renegotiate our relationship with our needs and with those who fulfill them.

Developmentally the oral character is thought to arise from roughly the first year of life. This is a time when a baby's needs are very great and their resources for meeting these needs are still very small, and so the baby is very dependent on their caregiver. Food, rest, play, comfort, love, warmth, and contact all need to be provided by the caregiver. At the beginning of this period, the baby has to rely on the caregiver reading the baby's needs correctly; toward the end of the period, the baby will usually have developed ways of communicating needs more reliably. If the caregiver doesn't meet the baby's needs, or fails to read them reasonably accurately, the baby will conclude that they have no right to need anything. This central tragedy in a young life usually has one of two consequences: either there will be a huge need inside the person that is ever-present and can never be completely fulfilled (this is called the "collapsed oral character") or the person will decide not to need anything and will spend their life making sure they don't need anything (this is called the "compensated oral character").

Either of these options will leave a legacy of anger and resentment—anger at the world for not providing for the needs of a baby who was, after all, not able to provide for themself. Sometimes the anger is retroflected at the baby who was so needy. This happens especially if the neediness is also experienced as shameful. Anger at the baby may also be the result of identification with a caregiver who reacted with anger to a baby's expression of need. We can think of a mother who is not coping well with sleep deprivation and an unsettled and grizzly baby, who expresses her anger with the baby, or of a family where there are too many needy children and not enough food or attention or love to go around, and the parents attack the neediness in their children.

Just from this simple description it is easy to see that ignored children are going to have injuries going back to this period. Ignored children have experienced that their needs have not been adequately met. Sometimes this has created so much hardship for the child that they have done their best not to even perceive their needs. This will then lead to a situation in which the ignored child doesn't know what they need. Usually one need that the person will still try to fulfil is the need for an attachment relationship. So the ignored child will spend a large part of their life looking for a parent, an authority figure, or somebody to look after them and keep them safe. Often this is combined with a yearning to belong with a group or tribe that the person can identify with and in this way fulfil their attachment needs. The complete suppression of any needs can result in the lack of a sense of self and a lack of direction in life, because this is what needs are for: to help us become aware of where there is a beneficial environment for us and start us moving in that direction.

Physically, the typical oral character presents as rather underdeveloped, as if the body expresses the lack of being fed enough. The whole body can lack vitality, leaving perhaps only the eyes to reach out with longing. It can give an impression of being about to collapse from the unsustainability of the effort. Contact with the earth is often poor, making the business of everyday life indeed hard work. Often oral characters look younger than their age, as if they have not entirely grown up. They are usually outgoing and contactful rather than withdrawn and often very sociable or even clingy.

If a person has been ignored in the first year of their life, invariably their needs will also have been ignored. At the very least this will create a working model of the world as a place where needing something is a waste of time. You either go and fulfill your own need, or you do without; at any rate the world will not respond to your need in a positive way. That would be the basic position. We almost never find this in a person. Instead, for most ignored children there seems to be a further interpretation that there is something bad about either the ignored child as a person or about the need. Either the child thinks, "I don't get my needs met, so I must be a bad person who doesn't deserve it," or the child thinks, "I don't get my needs met so needing must be bad." If the "bad" is located largely in the person, the resulting character style will be more schizoid; if the "bad" is located in the need, the resulting character style will be more oral. We can see that the former creates a more pervasive and more generalized shame; the latter creates a lot of shame and internal persecution centered around the person's needs.

We find in both oral and schizoid characters that the internal child who feels so bad often gets vilified by the more adult part of the client. We can understand this as an identification with, or loyalty toward, the parents whose behavior gave rise to the bad feelings in the first place. From the point of view of the parent, it is the needs that are the problem, and if it wasn't for the child's neediness, all would be well. For the child, to follow in this belief may rescue of a part of their personality (everything that isn't needy), but it will make the healing of the wound, with or without psychotherapy, more difficult. This is because anything that prevents a person from feeling compassion toward their own suffering will act as a resistance to change. Undoing such internal *knots* is the slow, unspectacular business of long-term psychotherapy.

I mention these knots (which are a general feature of all neurotic symptoms) in this particular chapter because I have found that oral characters are prone to some very therapy-proof types of dynamics (Stauffer, 2005). I believe this is because the typical oral defenses create such a very successful and very culturally acceptable fantasy of how we should all be that it is almost impossible to give it up and settle for what feels like much less. Especially the fantasy of not needing anything and of being independent and self-sufficient is a pervasive idealization in our culture of how people should be. If we no longer aspire to this ideal, we need to accept fallibility, weakness, and dependency on others as part of normal life, and this is very difficult for people in a culture where such qualities are attached to massive shame and perhaps danger. Particularly in persons who also have a history of early caregivers being invasive or abusive, the avoidance of needs and dependency acquires an additional urgency. Both for individuals and for our society, it is sad that the experience of interdependence, which paints a realistic picture of how human beings really are, doesn't seem to gain much general acceptance.

Most theoreticians differentiate between the "collapsed" and the "compensated" oral character (Totton & Edmondson, 1988). The compensated oral character is typically a compulsive caregiver, and for women especially, compulsive caregiving is a very successful defense. My work with Pearl may illustrate this:

It is so easy to tell Pearl that she needs to look after herself better. Everybody says so. When she feels very stressed and overwhelmed, she can even enjoy other people's solicitude. The feeling never lasts long. Invariably her concern for others returns, together with her fear that she is being too selfish, or bad, or taking something away from others. The thought of her loved ones' suffering is unbearable.

Time after time, she stops looking after herself again and devotes all her energy the well-being of those around her.

Her fear of what will happen if she stops caregiving is allied to the vicarious gratification she gets from it. It is also allied to a very early and largely wordless terror of what price she will have to pay for getting some of her needs met: her experience is that her mother reacted very grumpily when she had to "waste her time" on Pearly because Pearl needed something. Getting her needs met therefore came with punishment in the form of Mother's hostility and criticism.

To add a further factor stabilizing the caregiving behavior, Pearl has built her identity on being the loving and empathic mother who will never be like her own mother and will never make her children feel as terrible as she felt as a child. This has become a central pillar of her sense of who she is, and asking her to change it is like asking her to become a different person. Just interpreting and elucidating this internal dynamic of hers is not sufficient to allow it to change, because way too much depends on it being in place. The shift in the dynamic will be very slow and require many new resources and new ways of being in the world.

The only therapeutic strategy that I can think of is to discuss with her how much she needs to suffer, in her own internal judgment, in order to be allowed to have something good for herself. Because this allows for nuances in between the black-and-white dilemma of either caring for herself or caring for others, I feel that there may be some therapeutic hope in it. At least it provides us with some instances in which she has accepted care from others (and seeking therapy with me was initially one such instance) and it has been a good experience. It allows us to build a language for the problem that does not put too much pressure on her, and that both signals to her my understanding of her difficulty and my hope that we can make some changes. Gradually it also creates a little distance between Pearl and "the problem."

Hypo-Responsiveness and Developmental Deficits

Bodynamic Analysis is the only psychotherapeutic modality I know that has developed a clinically useful model of hypo-responsiveness (Macnaughton, 2004; Marcher & Fich, 2010). The term hypo-responsiveness derives from the response of a muscle that lacks tone, or is hypotonic (or under-toned). A hypotonic muscle will respond to almost any challenge not by tensing and thus rising to the challenge, but by the opposite: it will slacken further, thus giving up and resigning itself to losing or avoiding the challenge. Most people have some muscles in their bodies that are under-toned in this way, muscles the person feels have no strength, which have never been developed or whose development has been relinquished following extreme trauma. Such muscles can exist alongside others that are the opposite, over-toned or hypertonic, as well as muscles with good tone. There is thought to be a functional unity between such hypo-responsive muscles and developmental deficits. It is important to note that the pattern of hypo-response, or giving up instead of engaging and attempting to rise to challenge, does not only occur in muscle but also in every other system of the body and, importantly, in the mind.

Merete Holm Brantbjerg has developed this concept further, focusing on developing a methodology for working with hypo-states in both the muscular system and the autonomic nervous system. Her focus is on the impact of such hypo-states on physical and psychological functioning, and how to negotiate this impact (Holm Brantbjerg, 2012). Hypo-states are very often found in ignored children. Hypo-responsiveness seems to be a typical sequel of emotional neglect, and we can perhaps understand why: neglect creates minds that lack resources and also lack good experiences of overcoming challenges. Instead, for ignored children, life is a continuous struggle in which they are typically only just able to hold their own by exerting themselves as hard as they can. When a challenge comes along, it can only be perceived as adding to this burden and may overwhelm the person. They simply will not have the resources needed for engaging with a challenge in any other way than by giving up.

The relevance of this theory for the subject of emotional neglect is that the hypo-responsiveness is embodied and occurs in a functional identity between the skeletal musculature and the psychological functioning. Moreover, a clear developmental origin of hypo- versus hyper-responsiveness is being postulated. This is derived from the gradual increase of voluntary control over the skeletal musculature that children acquire during the first 3 years of life or so. This gradual acquisition parallels the main stages of psychological development that children undergo during the same period and indeed happens in close interaction with it. This view of child development is called psychomotor development. The increase of muscular control that happens as a result of normal bodily growth enables a child to explore and grow into new movements, new skills, and new facets of life experience; at the same time, these new experiences imbue the newly controlled muscles and new movements with life and meaning.

The growing into new motoric capabilities happens in developmental stages. Each stage will have an early phase in which the movement is quite tentative and may not succeed every time and a late phase in which the movement is repeated many times until the child appears to have had enough and loses interest. If a movement is discouraged early in the appropriate developmental stage, the result will be a hypo-responsive muscle, representing a giving up and later avoidance of the movement. This scenario is likely to represent the functional equivalent of a developmental deficit. On the other hand, if a movement is discouraged in the late phase, the result may be a hypertonic muscle representing an often frustrated inability to let go or an ambivalent or conflicted attitude toward the movement. This latter possibility is likely to represent the functional equivalent of a developmental conflict. The assumption that hypo-responsiveness derives from early injuries and hyper-responsiveness derives from late ones does not hold completely true, because when something extremely dramatic happens in the late phase of a developmental stage, a child can respond by retreating entirely from this developmental stage and falling back onto an earlier stage, thus resulting in hypo-responsiveness with regard to this developmental stage (Holm Brantbjerg, personal communication, 2019). For the purposes of this text, we can assume that ignored children are often not encouraged to seek new experiences and often end up fearing them. Therefore injuries early in developmental stages with resulting hypo-responsive muscle groups will be common among those who were ignored children.

Again, I repeat the point that most classical psychotherapeutic theories and practices have been constructed for issues that are hypertonic, such as internal conflicts, issues that a person is unable to let go of, or impulses that have got stuck in the person and are pressing for completion. The kinds of issues that result in hypo-responsiveness are far less well described in the literature: the never-attempted skills, the hopelessly unattainable visions, the thoughts that seem utterly foreign to a person, the relinquished potentials.

The connection between a child's development and the skeletal musculature in the adult gives us a very elegant means of conceptualizing child development in a way that makes it accessible to direct experience in adult life. As a consequence, if we explore movements and muscle groups that are hypo-responsive, we may gain access to the experience of being neglected and ignored by our caregivers. More importantly, we can also experience the movements and muscle groups that are well developed and gain a sense of being better resourced from such an exploration. Thus the body can serve as a vehicle for developing the psychophysical functions that have not been developed in early childhood.

Holm Brantbjerg (2020) calls her approach relational trauma therapy. It has a lot to teach us about hypo-responsiveness in general. Hypo-responsive areas of the body are normally difficult to have a sense of ownership of and to feel as a part of the self. Trying to inhabit such areas of the body may be difficult or even create a sense of discomfort, nausea, or dizziness. A key concept for working with this difficulty is *dosing down*, the gentle activation of the musculature in a hypo-responsive part of the body in such small doses that the musculature does not feel overwhelmed and fatigued. The following example will illustrate this approach:

> I get Mortimer to try some muscle-tensing exercises as part of his anxiety management. The approach has the advantage of giving him something fairly structured to do and something that creates an immediate state change, that calms him and connects him to here and now. It also builds a habit in him of making use of the feelings and sensations in his body to teach him how to discriminate what is good for him and what is not. Isometric-type muscle-tensing exercises need to be done in such a way that they feel pleasant if they are to be effective. We can thus use these exercises to mobilize some good feelings and an atmosphere of fun between us as we try out different ways of creating a little tension in his muscles. I simply provide some resistance to his movements, and he lets me

know which of these movements feel nice to him and which ones don't. As we do this, I notice that it is fairly easy for me to feel which muscles respond with some pleasure to the challenge and which ones don't. At first, he wants to "be good" and focus on the muscles that don't feel strong. I have to encourage him actively to show me how strong he is and really let me feel the strength in his muscles. Gradually he begins to enjoy letting me see and feel his strength, and how big and powerful this makes him feel. At the end of 15 minutes, we are both a little breathless but warm, happy, and present in the room, and he looks for all the world as if he had grown half an inch.

Another important lesson that we learn from relational trauma therapy is that hypo-responsiveness is part of most traumatic experiences and most traumatic memories. As our habitual functioning fragments under the influence of an overwhelming experience, we may consciously focus on those parts of the experience that retain some sense of control and agency. States of collapsing, giving up, and surrendering to psychological or physical death, of not wanting to be there and therefore numbing ourselves or leaving our bodies, are also part of most traumatic experiences; just like the incomplete actions directed at saving our lives, they remain alive in the body and in the psyche (Holm Brantbjerg, 2012). If we are to complete traumatic memories, we will at some point have to address these low-energy states, even if most of us feel distinctly uncomfortable sitting with despair, depression, helplessness, or deep resignation and preparation for death.

Yet, given that everybody is a mixture of hyper- and hypo-responsive parts, we can also assume that every ignored child will have resources that can be developed and used as seedlings for new personality traits. The following vignette may illustrate this:

One day, Olivia comes in feeling particularly depressed. She will have to undergo a medical procedure and is secretly convinced that she is seriously ill and will soon die, having lived a very impoverished life that failed to give her any real fulfilment. Everything feels empty and pointless, and she is very collapsed in hopelessness. I sense that she has gone somewhere that feels very early, like a very young child who is sure she is about to die. As I feel myself being pulled into the same hopelessness and depression, I remind myself that this self-state is not all there is in Olivia. In fact, she has fallen prey to an old memory, and it is indeed a long time ago that there was any reality to the way she feels right now.

I feed this insight back to her. She finds it hard to engage with me, because her feelings are so powerful and feel very much here and now, and she cannot believe that I might have a point. I encourage her to breathe a little and sit with the thought that this happened a long time ago and she survived. Suddenly she lifts her head up and looks at me with a beseeching look in her eyes, and says, "It's true, isn't it? I did survive?" There is a question mark in her voice. I repeat a couple of times that yes, she did survive. Then I add, "You are a survivor." The word completely galvanizes her. Her spine straightens, her head lifts further, and a smile spreads over her face. "I am a survivor," she repeats several times. For the rest of this session, I just help her anchor this thought in the muscles of her back and legs, which give her strength, and I also help her integrate the new identity as a survivor into her inner life. It takes some months for the felt sense of being a survivor to become completely familiar. During this time her whole identity undergoes a considerable shift. She becomes less disempowered and more able to actively make her life better, and I observe a big surge of new and more resourced life in her.

One of the more valuable contributions of relational trauma therapy is the distinction between low energy in the autonomic nervous system (ANS) and low energy in the musculature. Many psychotherapists these days are used to observing the state of their clients' ANS and may be able to spot when a client shows signs of freezing, which suggests a hypo-activity that needs to be brought into some sort of window of tolerance. However, most therapists are not used to observing the state of the client's musculature (and sometimes the connective tissues as well), where a low energy state leads to being easily overwhelmed with anxiety. Such clients do not suffer from low energy in their ANS—on the contrary, they may feel extremely anxious or panicked. The combination of high energy in the ANS and low energy in the musculature results in a very easily overwhelmed person who struggles to contain their feelings. On the other hand, many people live in the opposite state, having good muscles that are able to contain very powerful feelings, so that on the face of it they look very stable and high-functioning. Yet this appearance may be deceptive if the person has learned just to bury their anxiety under strong muscles rather than to regulate it. In that case a person will be rather vulnerable to burning out. Ignored children occur in both of these categories, and if we look at the examples I am using in this book, we can say that Mortimer, Olivia, and Pearl are high energy in the ANS; Mortimer is also low energy in the musculature, whereas Olivia and Pearl are less so. Norman has a tendency to high energy in the musculature and low energy in the ANS.

Relational trauma therapy has developed a complex and exhaustive repertoire of movement-based exercises designed to enhance resources for clients with low-energy states. This is called resource-oriented skills training (ROST) and is available from the relevant website (Moaiku, 2019). I do not imagine that readers of this book should start using these exercises with their clients; rather, I have included a brief summary of the work here because it is to my knowledge the best approach currently available for working with such states and such clients, and it is therefore an important theory for therapists who work with ignored children and with developmental deficits.

CHAPTER 4

Neuroscientific Contributions Toward Understanding Ignored Children

At this point I want to change gears and present some of the evidence from scientific research that supports my understanding of how ignored children function and what they are struggling with (for reviews see De Bellis, 2005; De Bellis et al., 2009; Hildyard & Wolfe, 2002; Joseph, 1999; Perry, 2002; Sciarrino et al., 2018; Shipman et al., 2005). I will focus on what seems useful to me and serves to promote my own ability to resonate with the experience of clients who were ignored children, which I feel is central for all therapists who want to work with this client group.

One of the few studies that have specifically looked at neglected children finds that these children have a particular bias in recognizing emotions on the faces of others (Lopez-Duran et al., 2013). On the whole, they recognize threatening and angry faces more easily than happy and loving ones. It is as if they see the world through a filter of their own expectations of being met with hostility and anger. This to me illustrates powerfully the consequences of neglect: when a child feels loved, the world is friendly and benign and a good place to be. However, when a child does not feel loved, the world does not merely become neutral: it becomes hostile. This is further supported by the finding that neglect creates a more reactive amygdala (Bogdan et al., 2012). The amygdala is part of the primitive survival system of the brain, and we can assume that having a reactive amygdala means being primed to react with fear to many situations that might not in themselves be particularly dangerous. A reactive amygdala therefore promotes the sense of living in a hostile world. This may go some way to explaining that ignored children tend to become withdrawn and psychologically implode into loneliness.

First I will delineate what we know about affect regulation in early infancy and how it shapes the personality of the child in later life. If we accept the centrality of affect regulation in child development, it follows of necessity that we will be struck by how disastrously children will be affected by malfunctions of this process. I will then go on and take a closer look at the autonomic nervous system (ANS), which is a central player in affect regulation. Observation of the physical signs of ANS activity is an astonishingly versatile and powerful tool to help us work with anxious people and to find ways of getting a taste of their experience. I will devote a separate section to the polyvagal theory by Stephen Porges and in particular to his work on the social engagement system, which powerfully argues that if ignored children can shift from experiencing other people as the problem to experiencing other people as the solution, their healing process will be greatly enhanced.

After this, I will look at three more specialized areas: The first of these is shame and the different insights that we have gained about it by various authors. The second is parentification and compulsive caregiving. I take my understanding of this largely from the work of Louis Cozolino. And finally, I will discuss the available evidence that suggests that ignored children may be more prone than others to physical illness, and possibly to somatizing, throughout their lives.

Neuroscience of Early Development and Affect Regulation

In the last 20 years or so, several neuroscientists, some of whom also have a background in psychotherapy, have made a beginning on the project of trying to bring together the two disciplines and create some correlations between what we call the mind, which belongs in the domain of psychotherapy, and the brain, which belongs in the domain of neuroscience. Allan Schore is one of these, and his specialty is early brain development and what this means in terms of a person's psychological functioning. It is from his work that we have gained a clearer view of the importance of the early mother-infant interactions that are scarce or absent in ignored children. This allows us to extrapolate how the emotional functioning of ignored children may be affected by such a lack (Gerhardt, 2004; Hart, 2008; Schore, 1994, 2003).

Schore makes the point that the interactions between mother and child allow the infant's expressions to be mirrored by the mother and in turn mirror her affects in what is basically a process of reentry. Colwyn Trevarthen (1993) has demonstrated that infants are really interested in this process and will mirror what they see within minutes after birth. We can imagine that in such a way the two brains of caregiver and infant go into resonance with each other, and it is easy to speculate that this resonance creates a sense of emotional closeness and being seen and understood. Crucially, it also allows the infant's brain to develop its own resources for handling affects, and depending on the maturity of the mother's affect-regulation skills, the infant can learn more or less mature and sophisticated skills for managing feelings from early in life.

The development of affect regulation predates the cognitive development of children substantially and takes place mostly in the first 2 years of life. This is a time when the brain develops very rapidly and new areas of the brain, particularly parts of the cerebral cortex, gradually come online. We can picture this development by imagining that the brain is being composed of layers, rather like an onion. For most researchers it seems to make sense to distinguish three concentric layers as follows:

- At birth, we only have the innermost layer of the onion available to regulate our affects—mainly the amygdala-based networks that are programmed for survival and operate in a crude, all-or-nothing manner. This means that very young infants don't have many options for affect regulation except to avoid disturbing stimuli, numb their own feelings, or perhaps freeze and play dead.
- The second layer gets added on during the first 6 months of a baby's life. This comprises networks centered around the cingulate gyrus and allows more differentiation in response and more contact with others including experiences of pleasure, leading to first smiles and moments of shared fun.
- Finally, the third layer starts to come online by about 10–12 months. It consists of networks centered around the orbitofrontal cortex, and we have here the beginnings of a capacity to self-reflect and to adapt responses in a considered manner to the environment (Stauffer, 2010).

I suspect that it is predominantly the second stage of this development that goes missing in ignored children and sometimes partly the third. The first is active at birth and therefore always available, but it is a very primitive system of self-regulation aimed purely at surviving, all black-and-white without any shades of gray, and prone to overreacting. The processes it uses for the purpose of self-regulation can be very unpleasant to experience, involving possibly extreme fear and rage or freezing and dissociation. These processes are there to assure the physical survival of the individual. They are not really capable of taking into account the existence of other people, and therefore a person who only functions on this level will look like an asocial and very paranoid person. This level of functioning is sometimes called the *reptilian brain*, suggesting that if it was the only functioning available to us, we would lack essential humanity.

Processes that become activated in the second stage of development are by comparison much more interpersonal and attachment-related. It is here that we can see ignored children missing out. If somebody learns very early on that reaching out for comfort and help is not a good idea, they will quickly stop doing it, and all the emotional circuitry in the brain that is associated with the formation of interpersonal bonds will remain underdeveloped. Being comforted, feeling close and cozy, being happy to be oneself, or having fun, are all going to be experiences that an ignored child doesn't have. They will not learn to make use of others for regulating their affects, and therefore other people remain a source of worry and fear rather than a source of comfort and joy.

In addition, during this time there is an opportunity to learn that excitement is not only a bad experience, but also that it can be fun and can include the shared experiences that give life its joy and tastiness. Such good experiences increase the range of tolerable excitement that a person will have available to them without undue distress. For children who struggle to regulate their affects without having a good range of regulatory possibilities available to them, affect regulation may always remain a difficult and arduous task, and excitement of any kind may remain a deeply negative experience to be avoided at all costs. We can easily imagine how this type of mechanism lays the foundation for an attitude toward life that avoids being fully alive in order not to risk difficult and possibly unmanageable feelings (see also De Bellis et al., 2002; Maheu et al., 2010; Norman et al., 2012).

The third layer represents a further development toward more sophisticated self-regulation strategies. Development is hierarchical in the sense that each developmental stage builds on the attainments of the previous one. We can therefore assume that if in a developmental sequence there is a stage partly or wholly missing, there will be serious consequences of this lack in all the later stages.

Human beings are amazingly versatile and find ways of working around large holes in their brains. In my experience, in ignored children the strategies associated with the third layer are often overdeveloped and may be used to compensate for the gaps in the second layer. There may be, for example, a strong ability to rationalize and reassure anxieties using rational thought, to observe what other people do and learn from these observations, or to deduce rules for behavior. Often in ignored children these strategies have a fragile quality, as if the person has to carefully think their way through the process step by step, rather than doing it intuitively as an implicit process. We also find that ignored children may be able to function adequately for a while—until they are of school age, or until puberty, or into their early 20s—and eventually come to the end of their tether and develop symptoms of mental ill-health, seemingly in response to quite a minor event or even without an obvious precipitating event. To my mind, this points to the fragility and unsustainability of their mental and emotional functioning and represents a serious form of burnout. It underpins my impression that the type of traumatization that ignored children suffer from resembles more the symptoms of burnout than symptoms of abuse.

Let me use a session with Pearl as an example of the fragile quality of the third-layer defenses of an ignored child. We are talking about her daughter and how she often tells Pearl off for "fussing" and "being invasive and controlling." On the one hand, Pearl can see that this is probably true. On the other hand, she is completely driven to keep trying to control her daughter's behavior, which she sees as dangerous and therefore intolerable. To stop doing this is unthinkable; she thinks she would die of fright if she were to do that. So in her mind there is an absolute necessity to control something that, in the final analysis, she cannot control (her daughter's behavior). At the same time, she thinks of her daughter's impulsive behavior as the problem. She thus locates the problem as "out there" and doesn't feel able to question the adaptiveness of her own response or her own judgment; rather she defends with great eloquence and persuasiveness how absolutely necessary and nonnegotiable her controlling behavior is.

It is this eloquence that gives me the hint that I am on the receiving end of something not entirely rational. I begin to understand that Pearl has dropped into a much younger ego state where she identifies with the daughter and really feels herself in danger. I mirror this back to her: "It seems to me that you have gone to an old terror about what could happen to a young girl in a big, dangerous world. That must make it very difficult for you to respond with any kind of detachment." In this way, I manage to get Pearl back into a more adult ego state. She is grateful that I have understood the terrible pressure that she experiences all the time. We spend some time acknowledging the experiences that she had when she felt unprotected and at risk as a teenager. Gradually she can see that being under this much pressure has made it impossible for her to see that there might be more adaptive ways of dealing with her parenting difficulties. The insight that her seemingly rational thinking is actually very heavily colored by a much more primitive fear makes it possible for us to explore this state of affairs a little more. She is eventually able to find some differences between her own teenage self and her daughter and begin to trust the daughter's resources a little more. I affirm that after all, her daughter has a loving and very attentive mother to help her cope with difficulties.

We have increasing evidence that the absence of good affect-regulatory experience and loving contact with caregivers produces changes in the brain structure and chemistry. For example, it is thought that early neglect may lead to a resistance of the brain to cortisol through initial overexposure, and in turn this resistance to cortisol numbs the range of emotional experience available to the person, thus making them more vulnerable to stressful events (Gerhardt, 2004). We learn from this that the absence of love does not produce a neutral world but a hostile and stressful one, and starting out in this manner means that a person's resources for dealing with subsequent life experiences are curtailed, and so the damage keeps getting worse.

The Autonomic Nervous System

The autonomic nervous system (ANS) forms part of the efferent (motor) branch of the peripheral nervous system. In this capacity, it acts as the transmitter of commands from the brain to all tissues and organs of the body. The activity of the ANS thus leads to physical changes in the body as a function of the changes in the way the brain experiences life on a moment-by-moment basis. From the activity of the ANS it is not usually possible to tell which part of the brain, or layer, a particular command is coming from—all commands from the brain will be transmitted to the body via the ANS.

What gives the ANS its great usefulness for psychotherapists is the fact that changes in ANS activity can be experienced physically in one's own body and observed in the body of another person. Therefore for psychotherapists, tracking signs of ANS activity in themselves and in their clients is a powerful tool for fine-tuning both the quality of a relationship (particularly relational safety) and also the general state of arousal including anxiety (Carroll, 2001, 2005, 2009; Levine, 1997; Rothschild, 2017; Stauffer, 2009;). This gives therapists the option of keeping clients within their window of tolerance and avoiding re-traumatization (Siegel, 1999).

Traditional neuroscience teaches about two branches of the ANS: the sympathetic branch that mediates broadly excitatory processes, and the parasympathetic branch that mediates more inhibitory processes. In terms of subjective experience, excitatory processes include feelings of excitement, fear, anger, and disgust. Inhibitory processes include feelings of calm, contentment, sadness, and shame. Most of the emotions that we are all familiar with are mediated by both branches to varying degrees. This somewhat limiting view of ANS activity has been challenged by a number of authors, both on neurophysiological grounds and on grounds of clinical practice. In recent years, the simple model of linear adjustments in the state of excitement/inhibition in the body has been replaced with a more sophisticated concept of autonomic space that is more multidimensional and allows for more subtlety in subjective experience and for a wider range of possible somatic markers (Berntson et al., 1994).

In Chapter 3, I referred to the importance of the ANS in mediating cycles of emotional and embodied experience ("vasomotoric cycles"). In terms of ANS activity, this corresponds to an orderly progression of sympathetic activity followed by parasympathetic activity in such a way that the two branches initially inhibit and later activate each other.

It is typical for ignored children that such cycles of well-regulated ANS activity are not very strongly developed. A person who lacks confidence in their own ability to deal with states of high arousal will mostly try to keep life on an even keel and make sure that arousal remains as low as possible. In terms of vasomotoric cycles, we can assume that ignored children will try to keep them small in amplitude and may appear to cling to a state of rest. Sadly, this can be misread by others as an attempt to control, as cold superiority, or as inability to feel deeply.

The consequences for ignored children of this need to keep movements in the ANS small are very severe and may present a lifelong burden. We often find in ignored children a reduced ability to take risks and play for high emotional stakes: this happens especially when approval by important figures in their lives or contact with attachment figures is at stake. The terror of losing such tenuous bonds often leads ignored children to remain within the narrow confines of familiar self-regulatory resources and avoid seeking to widen their range of interpersonal activities. In this way, ignored children may be condemned to limit their opportunities for success both in their professional and in their social lives, as well as limiting the scope of therapeutic improvement of which they are capable.

In intimate relationships, it is a common fate for ignored children to be accused by their partners of being controlling and lacking spontaneity or depth of feeling. Ignored children with fragile interpersonal boundaries usually come off worst, because poor boundaries and brittle affect regulation both contribute to making relationships incredibly stressful and hard work. For these ignored children, the fear of other people may lead them to abstain from having relationships at all. It is my experience that when such clients present for therapy, they have a particularly painful experience: they will need to learn that the treatment for their lack of connection will be initially to strengthen their ability to remain separate and not become invaded by others who get close. This is completely counterintuitive for many and can be very hard to accept.

Over time I have spent quite a lot of sessions with Mortimer working on his boundaries. He can never quite believe that it could be a good idea for him to learn how to keep other people away—he is really uncertain whether he is entitled to do that. Being the compliant person he is, he politely agrees with me when I explain my reasons. However, I notice that when he is in company with another person, including me, he intuitively does the opposite. Clearly my injunctions don't reach to a level where he can understand the necessity for keeping himself safe. I try to work on his ability to regulate distance in a way that gives him some control over how close other people get without carrying a message that he should keep others at arm's length, but rather to emphasize that there may be an optimal distance and that he could find it moment by moment. This is only moderately successful. It seems to me that the main difficulty is that he is so strongly sucked into being identified with the other person that he just cannot keep enough of a hold on himself to even know how he feels, let alone think about how to feel better. For a long time, I continue to work on his boundaries and on his ability to return to himself. Typically, I will ask him to close his eyes and see what he notices inside himself, be that body sensations, emotions, impulses to move, and so on. I do this quite frequently during sessions, so that he shuttles back and forth between being focused on me and being focused on himself. I always get him to name what he notices, and when it seems to relate to something that just happened between us, I may gently draw his attention to that and invite him to find it interesting. Over a period of many months there is a slow improvement of his ability to remain in his own body. He also acquires an ability to create more connections between his internal state and external events. As this ability grows, he begins to notice how one-sided the balance between concern for other people's wellbeing and his own has always been, and he even voices a sense that this isn't quite fair. It seems to me that he is developing a stronger parental self that is wanting to look after him and keep him safe. This benign parental self has the power to give the necessity for safety equal weight with the need for identifying with the other. He describes it to me, "I feel that my thoughts are changing about what is okay for me. I used to think that anything bad that happened to me was fine, because I didn't deserve better, and so I could get hurt and it didn't matter. But now it seems to be just as important what I get out of a situation as whether I am pleasing the other person."

I want to say something about trauma at this point. From the point of view of the function of the ANS, we can say that trauma, as a state of being overwhelmed, represents a temporary inability of the ANS to function normally in emotional regulation (Rothschild, 1995). This may resolve itself in a matter of days or weeks following a traumatic event (and indeed does so in the majority of people who experience such an event). In some instances, it may lead to the installation of a new ego defense (as is common in developmental trauma). However, in a proportion of cases it persists and will show up as hyperarousal in the ANS of a person. Such signs of hyperarousal or post-traumatic stress can be spotted with a little practice both by clients themselves and by their therapists.

A way of conceptualizing the state of being overwhelmed is to look at the way that the sympathetic and parasympathetic nervous systems regulate each other: At low activity, both inhibit the other, whereas at high activity, both activate each other. In normal life this works very well: at rest, when sympathetic activity increases in response to an outer event, there comes a point at which the sympathetic nervous system starts to upregulate the parasympathetic. The parasympathetic then initiates a downregulation of the sympathetic, thus ensuring that sympathetic activity is limited and does not become uncontainable.

In this model it is easy to understand a state of overwhelm: it is generally initiated by extremely high activity in the sympathetic nervous system. This high activity upregulates the parasympathetic that is supposed to inhibit the sympathetic, thus restoring calm. When a situation is too frightening or carries on being frightening for too long, this fails to work, and parasympathetic activity also increases more and more. The end result is that both branches of the ANS will be at maximum activity, leading to a clinical picture that may well be a composite of both types of symptoms and represents an experience that cannot be integrated. States of dissociation, shock, numbness, or otherwise altered consciousness can all result from this pattern of activity in the ANS. Certainly the brain as a whole will no longer be in a state in which normal thought or normal processing of experience is possible. Physically, it may be possible to observe such states by spotting a mixture of symptoms of high sympathetic activity and symptoms of high parasympathetic activity (e.g., a pale face and bright red ears; or a calm voice and a racing heart, etc.). Therapists should not rely on this type of observation, though, and it is best to ask the client what they are aware of in their bodies if in doubt.

The advantage of this way of thinking is that we can easily imagine how difficult it is to calm such a state of the ANS. Ordinary, everyday calming by increasing parasympathetic activity clearly will not work here, and it seems more likely that the sympathetic activity will need to be reduced first in order to allow normal regulation to resume. This means that the perceived threat will need to subside and a measure of safety will need to be reestablished—in agreement with empirical findings from clinical practice (Levine, 1997; Rothschild, 2000).

We can see from this simple model how clients who were ignored children may be more vulnerable to traumatic events than others, by bearing in mind that the ability of their parasympathetic nervous system to downregulate the sympathetic nervous system is not very strongly developed. Therefore, when there is a powerful activation of the sympathetic nervous system by an external event, the activity of the whole autonomic nervous system may more easily increase into the domain where normal regulation is no longer possible.

Polyvagal Theory and the Social Engagement System

Stephen Porges' polyvagal theory (2001) represents an enormously useful elaboration on the more traditional thinking about the ANS. Its main feature is the division of the parasympathetic nervous system into two different systems, the dorsal vagal complex (DVC) and the ventral vagal complex (VVC). This division turns out to correspond to two distinct and clinically meaningful states of *stillness*. Under the influence of the DVC, the organism becomes immobilized in a way that corresponds to freezing, quite likely in terror or dissociation. On the other hand, under the influence of the VVC, the organism calms and comes to rest in a way that feels pleasant, relaxing, and peaceful. Moreover, the VVC is also termed the social engagement system and constitutes the main agent by which infants and small children learn to find safety and happiness in contact with others. We can call it the mediator of bonding, and this is as true in adults as in children.

According to the polyvagal theory, the ANS thus consists of three branches, not two. Phylogenetically and ontogenetically the oldest is the DVC. Then we have the sympathetic nervous system (SNS), and finally the VVC as the most recent branch of the ANS. It also seems likely that while the DVC and the SNS are fully active at birth, the social engagement system is only potentially available and needs to be developed in contact with early caregivers. We can assume that the social engagement system is the most vulnerable branch of the ANS.

The polyvagal theory implies that we have two ways of inhibiting a state of excessive excitement in our bodies and minds: we can either use fear to stop moving and become quiet as a mouse and attempt to be invisible (and this uses the DVC); or we can seek out proximity to another person to make us feel safe and at peace (and this uses the VVC). Once we have experienced these two different states as small children, they become internalized to the point that we can put ourselves into the state of mind that corresponds to being with a safe person without them being actually physically present: there is now in our minds a blueprint of calm that is derived from our early experiences of being held safely and is mediated largely by the social engagement system.

If, on the other hand, we have not experienced being held safely when very small; or if that experience has been patchy and interrupted before we had time to internalize it properly, then it may not be reliably available to us and we may have to resort to using the DVC to help downregulate the SNS. If we habitually use the DVC in this way, we remain very vulnerable to stress, because high activity in the DVC itself signals to the body and to the brain that we live in a dangerous and stressful environment. Clearly this will affect our physical and emotional health. It is important to realize that, as is usual in complex biological systems, too much is more dangerous than too little, and therefore a state of great excitement absolutely needs to be downregulated in order to preserve the safety and optimal functioning of the organism as a whole.

I believe that this accounts for the observation that in the absence of good contact, the world is not experienced as neutral but turns hostile. Downregulating activity in the sympathetic nervous system is not optional but needs to happen somehow; if all a person has available is the DVC, then they will experience danger and threats at every turn. I believe that such experiences shape to a substantial degree the inner world of ignored children.

Having three branches of the ANS instead of two greatly enlarges the range of different autonomic states that we can think of, in which there are different levels of activity of all three branches present simultaneously. The polyvagal theory therefore makes it much easier to visualize how different affective experiences might represent different states of activity in the ANS.

We can use the polyvagal theory to reinterpret what constitutes a state of shock, or trauma: It looks like the central component is powerful activity in the DVC. To be sure, we can assume that the sympathetic will also be activated. However we now have a useful conceptualization for the state of freeze (which may involve a greater or lesser extent of dissociation) in the dorsal vagal complex, together with the idea of a very old and primitive lifesaving device. The thought that in a life-threatening situation the brain ditches all the regulation strategies it has acquired and resorts to the earliest programs of survival makes a lot of sense for many people. It may be added that this state of the ANS can go with more or less tension in the musculature. If most of the muscles tense up under the influence of the DVC, the result will be a state of tonic immobility, or frozen stiffness, whereas if most of the muscles go limp in response to the DVC, the result will be a more collapsed state of utter surrender to what is happening (and potentially preparation for death). I have said more about this distinction in Chapter 3, in the section about relational trauma therapy.

Probably the most important question for anybody who experiences a state of shock or trauma is how to get out of it. Clearly, shocking and traumatizing events just happen and we cannot prevent them (although particularly adults who were ignored children seem to spend an awful lot of time and energy attempting to do this). Our nervous system has got mechanisms available for returning to normal and getting over shocking events, and in the majority of people who experience even a major disaster, these mechanisms act to restore normal functioning in a matter of days or weeks. We can speculate that the social engagement system plays a central role in many of these mechanisms—and indeed this is underpinned by finding that strong social networks are the best protection as well as the best therapy for states of shock and trauma (Sahar, Shalev & Porges, 2001). By looking at the profoundly traumatized state that is represented by a maximal activity in the DVC, we can also appreciate just how disabled people are who don't have a good and robust social engagement system. Among those people are, of course, ignored children (Powers, Ressler, & Bradley, 2009).

I want to also emphasize the disastrous consequences of the lack of joyful experiences in the company of others that leaves ignored children with a heavy burden of social anxiety, avoidance, and often stigmatization as oddballs or geeky loners. We can see how an absence of shared states of pleasure and fun early in life can easily generate an absence of reliance on the social engagement system as a go-to resource for self-regulation. Ignored children will instead have the expectation that excitement is difficult to manage and best avoided. This seems tragic in a world in which so much value is placed by most people on shared fun and noisy enjoyment in company. The inability to engage in such activities that many ignored children experience often adds considerably to their shame and their sense that they are somehow deficient, freakish, or inadequate.

There is now an increasing body of research on the social engagement system, characterizing in some detail the nerves involved (see for example Lim & Young, 2006). Porges also postulates a very interesting connection between the face, especially the area around the eyes, and the heart of a person, thus creating a scientific narrative for the common experience that loving eyes are one of the key ingredients that create a secure attachment and the potential for happiness (Porges, 2017). A colleague has framed the loving gaze of our primary caregiver as the event that "switches us on to life"—implying that once this has happened, everything else is much easier, and life becomes a fundamentally positive experience (J. Waterston, personal communication, 2019).

In psychotherapy, eye contact is a variable that can be adjusted to the therapeutic intention and to the aims of a therapeutic process as well as to the momentary needs of the client. When working with early material, many psychotherapists find that warm and benevolent eye contact is a helpful ingredient for successful work. Moreover, with some practice it is possible to use the quality of the gaze of clients as well as the quality of the eye contact between client and therapist as a source of information about the client's inner world and the representations of other people in their mind.

Eye contact is especially important to Norman. He often withdraws from me and will not make eye contact, thus showing me his feelings of depression and shame. Yet I notice, even in the darkest times of his suffering, that every week as he leaves my consulting room, he turns his head and seeks my face with his eyes, as if to cling on to me, just for a moment. I find this incredibly moving and see it as a sign of a tiny glimmer of hope in him. It seems like a vestige of his social engagement system that is still alive and ready to be activated again. This activation then happens in the integration and resolution phase of the therapy, when the shame has lost much of its importance and Norman and I have grown a lot of relational safety. In this safer phase he can make full eye contact again and feel good and at peace with himself while looking at me.

Shame

Shame is one of the experiences that all ignored children share, and it may make psychotherapy difficult. Some ignored children are so crippled by shame that psychotherapy is absolute torture, because everything the therapist says generates more shame that they can't process.

It needs to be understood that shame *per se* is an ordinary emotion that exists for a reason. Its primary function would seem to be to regulate an individual's place in the community. Shame may do this by making a person feel smaller when they are too big for the community and also by marginalizing individuals whose behavior does not serve the interests of the community. Marginalization exposes such individuals to danger and will hopefully enforce more conforming behavior. This function of shame presupposes an advanced emotional and cognitive development of the individual as well as situations that are easily remedied by corrected behavior. Clearly this is not the experience of those who suffer from pervasive and disabling shame; for them, shame is overwhelming and can never be redeemed. Therefore it seems sensible to distinguish between ordinary shame that can be processed and shame that cannot and overwhelms ordinary psychological functioning. The latter is often called toxic shame, and ignored children typically suffer from this type of shame.

They are not alone in this: in a time when narcissistic injuries are so common as to constitute a normopathy (Maaz, 2017), the inability to process shame is increasingly widespread, and destructive coping strategies such as passing shame on, or responding by attacking the person who is perceived as having delivered a shaming attack, are common. Nevertheless, it seems to me that in the work with ignored children, we are often dealing with shame that is especially pervasive and poisons the whole organism. Ignored children generally feel shame for not being able to do or know everything. Many feel extremely shamed when they stand out in any way and will go to enormous lengths in order to be invisible and blend in with their surroundings. This type of shame appears to relate to feeling exposed. Ignored children who have experienced an early rejection or abandonment by their primary caregivers will feel ashamed about being inadequate or unlovable. In addition, many ignored children feel ashamed of not being like others. Characteristics related to being introverted and shy generate huge amounts of shame. Finally, ignored children invariably feel ashamed of being so disabled by their shame and not able to just shrug it off.

All of these different types of shame can of course be felt by the same person, and they are often layered one on top of the other. It would appear, then, that ignored children respond to many different experiences with feelings of shame of varying intensity and toxicity. In general I find it helpful to address these different categories of shame separately. Some will respond to the increased resourcefulness and ego strength that is the result of good therapy; the most overwhelming ones may require trauma approaches such as eye movement desensitization and reprocessing (EMDR) or hypnosis.

An interesting categorization that is roughly along developmental lines has been put forward by Bracha Hadar (Hadar, 2008; Schultz-Venrath, 2018). She proposes a system of shame dimensions, as follows:

- *Archaic (malignant) shame* is the earliest and largely nonverbal, laid down as a somatic marker and about being unwanted. It can go back to before birth.
- *Primal shame* is associated with ruptures in attachment and develops in the attachment phase of development.
- *Recognition shame* is often manifested as self-consciousness and associated with the idea of looking at oneself as if with another's eyes. It develops somewhat later.
- *Sexual shame*, and generally shame that protects intimacy and has by some been called the shadow of sexuality, develops even later.
- *Social shame*, around exposing and embarrassing oneself, is the last to develop.

Hadar does not claim that this is a purely developmental sequence, and presumably it is possible to come up with slightly different taxonomies. What seems important to me is that if a child suffers from malignant shame from very early in life, all other shame dimensions are likely to be exacerbated and difficult to process. For my clients who have been ignored children, in particular recognition shame and social shame become conflated with the malignant shame and are generally not processable. In addition, ruptures in attachment are usually laden with a lot of shame and difficult to process.

The ability to process shame is generally developed around 10 to 24 months of age, and it is very much a function of the attachment relationship that a child finds themself in (Schore, 1994). It is therefore easy to recognize that if a child experiences strong shame well before that developmental period, this shame will not be processable and will be felt as traumatic. The presence of such traumatic shame may then make the normal acquisition of the ability to process shame difficult or impossible, and therefore subsequent shame may well just pile on top of this early unprocessed shame and make it all the more overwhelming. We can easily imagine this creating a cul-de-sac from which the person cannot escape.

In therapy, it may be difficult to recognize the presence of shame, because what shame does is create an impulse to hide. People who feel very ashamed will intuitively go to great lengths to hide their shame, and so it may be missed. It is tragic that the therapy for shame—its airing in the context of a safe and supportive relationship—is completely counterintuitive for shame-bound people. By avoiding having their shame seen, inadvertently they may be preventing their own healing.

Mortimer falls into this trap most often. His impulse to hide is so strong that he generally avoids shameful topics before he has had a chance to think. At first, my attempts to mirror back to him that he may be feeling ashamed seem to make the shame worse for being caught out. Other attempts to talk about shame seem equally unsuccessful, even if they probably provide some exposure therapy. Eventually I find an opportunity to allude, ever so casually, to the fact that shame makes us all want to hide and that this is really the worst thing for us, because as long as we hide, the shame can never get better. I say it in the kind of tone that suggests I am speaking of a well-known fact that he is familiar with. In response he laughs slightly sheepishly and says, "I've never thought of that before. It makes it easier."

Colwyn Trevarthen (2013) has made an important contribution to our understanding of shame in very small children. He has documented that from an early age, children like to initiate contact and often spontaneously reach out to engage another person in playful interaction.

When the other person does not respond, these children react with all the signs of severe shame. Such sequences recorded on film show what looks like a primitive shutdown mechanism in the ANS of the child, geared toward protecting the individual in this situation by recalibrating the organism to be oriented primarily inward. It is also visible in these films that this is a painfully abrupt process and may well be felt as an unpleasant shock by the child. It seems clear that if such sequences happen repeatedly, the child will almost invariably create a life script (or a "rule") around the dangers of reaching out to others and will become more and more reluctant to reach out for contact.

Trevarthen comments on this footage by putting the responsibility squarely on the adult in the interaction. Shame results when the adult doesn't understand. Or, slightly pointedly, "Shame is just other people's stupidity" (Trevarthen, 2013). His words point to a possible therapeutic intervention by taking the blame away from the child.

The scenario of reaching out in the absence of a response is probably the most benign one we can think of. Worse ones will include children who are the butt of their parents' critical, disappointed, and envious feelings and receive verbal attacks reflecting these attitudes. It seems likely that many mothers who experience postnatal depression treat their infants in quite a harsh fashion, often rejecting their attempts at making contact and blaming the child for their distress. Understandably, mothers who behave in such ways are in their turn deeply ashamed of themselves, thus making it difficult for their children to understand what happened to them early in life.

Another scenario is shame that may not be the person's own but somebody else's. This then becomes like a second-generation trauma: a distressing feeling for which the person has no narrative, because the feeling was somebody else's in the first place. The phenomenon is common among children with depressed mothers. We need to remember that children with highly insecure attachments are prone to resonating strongly with their caregivers—they generally become exquisitely attuned to their caregivers and will mirror the negative affect of their caregivers in an effort to create a safer relationship and better emotional regulation for themselves. This adaptive response also makes them more vulnerable to taking on negative feelings that aren't their own, such as shame. The shame then becomes more like a somatic marker than a specific memory and may persist lifelong. Another way of thinking about this mechanism is to view it as an identification with the aggressor—where the aggressor is also the main attachment figure (Schimmenti, 2012). This view helps us understand why it is so difficult to dissolve this shame in therapy: it is part and parcel of an extremely insecure attachment, and to let go of it would imply being able to let go, at least a little, of the attachment. I hope to have made the point by now that this is not an option for many clients who have been ignored children.

However, I do generally find it useful to suggest to clients that some of the shame they feel might not be theirs and to encourage them in the belief that they don't have to have it.

I do something similar one day with Olivia when she is particularly aware of how disgusting she feels she is. This is one of the deeper layers of her shame. The fear of being physically disgusting can poison most of her experiences. "I don't know where this comes from, but it's just deep within and I don't think I will ever be able to get rid of it. I am condemned to struggle with it all my life," she says. Responding to the first part of her statement I say, "I wonder if it was your adopted mother's disgust? She might have been preoccupied with her idealized fantasy that babies are all golden and sweet and had not quite allowed for the fact that they can also be rather messy and smelly at times. Might she sometimes have felt disgust and passed it on to you because it didn't fit her idealized image?" Olivia is very struck by this idea and starts to think more critically about what her mother might have experienced. This creates another step in the long process for her to separate from the adopted mother, to give up this terribly knotted attachment relationship and become a little more her own person.

Compulsive Caregiving

When I first read *The Neuroscience of Psychotherapy* by Louis Cozolino, my attention was grabbed by his description of what he calls pathological caretaking and which he sees as a form of narcissism:

> (. . . .) a reversal of the mirroring process during childhood. The narcissistic child's social brain and sense of self are not shaped by their own emerging emotions and sensibilities; rather, they are determined by their parents' own need for nurturance, attunement, and affect regulation. (Cozolino, 2002)

He alludes to a situation in which in an attachment relationship the caregiver does not respond to the child, does not mirror the child's feelings, and does not attune to the child's experience. He proposes that in that case the child's need for the attachment contact is so great that they will reverse the attachment relationship and start to mirror and attune to the caregiver. He concludes that this will leave the child with a lifelong sense of terrible inner emptiness that may never be filled. In Cozolino's opinion large tracts of implicit memory that would normally contribute to our sense of self remain confiscated by the identities of other people and thus can only ever form part of a false and compliant self, being essentially shut off from the person's deeper vital energy. The sense of self associated with the deep vitality of this person will remain wordless and unavailable to everyday experience and functioning and may feel totally empty.

Cozolino credits Alice Miller with the first description of this type of narcissism. It is sometimes called primary narcissism in recognition that it represents a profound loss of the person's sense of self and thus of the person's humanity, like all narcissistic wounds. Both Cozolino and Miller recognize that it arises at a very early age, long before the time when narcissistic wounds are thought to originate in traditional psychodynamic thinking (around 18 months of age). Both seem aware of what a terrible fate it is for an infant to be condemned to the inner emptiness and loneliness of a core self that had to be severely walled off, in an effort to preserve its identity, by a process that is so radical that there may be little hope of reversing it in a lifetime.

Miller's book, *The Drama of the Gifted Child* (1981), was a sensation in its time and made many people feel seen and understood in a profound way for the first time. I have found that when I speak to audiences about this reversal of the normal mirroring process, many respond in similar ways. Because from the beginning of their lives, the individuals affected in this way always had to be the "giver" and never the "receiver," they have never felt really loved. To have this deep wound seen by compassionate eyes creates great relief and comfort.

This process may be identical to, or at least closely related to, the process that more psychodynamic and attachment theorists call parentification—literally the process whereby a child is made into a parent. The impact of being part of such a reversed attachment relationship on the child's development will likely be very significant. If we think of a depressed mother, then we can see that a parentified child will mirror the mother's depression and almost certainly take it into themself. Indeed it has been found that the children of mothers with postpartum depression are at great risk themselves for depression later in life (Nikulina & Widom, 2013; Norman et al., 2012; Taillieu et al., 2016). It seems easy to postulate the route by which these children can inherit their mothers' depression: as far back as the 19th century, Charles Darwin observed that mimicking an affect will generate the feeling of it (Darwin, 1998). So the child of a depressed mother who mirrors her uninterested, sad, or miserable face will invariably end up feeling some of the mother's lack of interest, sadness, or misery.

If the mother is not depressed but fails to function as a parent for some other reason, parentified children will still lack the containment and safety that they need and will grow up having to look after themselves much too young. These children will later in life either embrace the responsibility of being a caregiver and parent to everybody around them, because this is the only way they know how to be and attain at least some social recognition; or they may dislike having to make choices and decisions and feel overburdened by any responsibility. In any case we can see the extra difficulty of having to be grown up too early when inside they feel empty—both factors make life hard work. Parentified children thus labor under two handicaps.

In the light of polyvagal theory, we can speculate that parentified children may miss out not only on finding safety and calm in proximity to a caregiver, but also on the experience of sharing fun and pleasure. Many parentified children grow up taking life a little too seriously and missing a blueprint for having fun in the security of a loving relationship in which it doesn't matter if you look foolish, there is no demand to do the right thing, and you are not having to make somebody happy, because you are both happy together. It is very easy to underestimate the importance of being playful in this way with another person. When it is absent, a child is likely to grow up always feeling a bit unloved and never quite good enough. They are also likely to grow up without confidence in their own ability to initiate the co-creation of good feelings with another person, which badly inhibits their social skills and confidence. On the whole, people can expect to be more vulnerable to stress and less confident if they have missed out on sharing fun with others early in life.

Many people are parentified in childhood, and not all of them grow up into compulsive caregivers. Most learn to receive care as well as give it. I have written about the phenomenology of this earlier (Stauffer, 2005). Nowadays I suspect that it usually takes a negative experience associated with receiving care in addition to being parentified to create a truly compulsive caregiver who can't seem to interact with others in any other way. I can think of clients who experienced being abused when vulnerable and in need, being vilified or shamed for being needy, seduced into inappropriate or invasive contact, or being left with the feeling that even when the parent was ostensibly looking after them there was still a "look-at-me-being-a-wonderful-parent" quality to the contact that made the interaction all about the parent and not about the child. At best, these clients have had mothers who were overworked and grumpy when a child needed something, because the mothers never got their own needs met.

In such a way the experience can get transmitted over generations, and many women, in particular, seem to come from long lines of parentified mothers who then use their own daughters to get some of their own needs gratified and to feel unconditionally loved. Over the course of the generations, the narrative can acquire additional twists such as contempt for people who have needs, or the heroism of those who don't have them, or the duty of good daughters to love and care for their mothers lifelong.

Part of the tragedy of this kind of childhood is that compulsive caregiving is such a successful coping strategy. Feeling powerful, strong, virtuous, altruistic, and deserving gratitude and appreciation are all among the potential benefits of it. In addition, the empathy with those whose needs compulsive caregivers look after may well give them a sense of vicarious gratification, and this may be as close as they ever get to real pleasure and fulfillment, especially with the finely-honed empathy skills of insecurely attached children. For many compulsive caregivers, the other side of the interaction, receiving care, is associated with powerlessness, weakness, victimhood, losing face, and often deep shame, thus further stabilizing the defense. It never seems to occur to compulsive caregivers that they expect others to be able to do something that they themselves cannot: to receive care with appreciation and gratitude.

Therapeutically I have found that compulsive caregiving is difficult to shift, presumably because it is such a successful defense and because the underlying experience so desperately needs to be defended against. There are also some typical difficulties that arise when clients try to change this pattern: they may feel themselves to be becoming more selfish, or may be accused of selfishness by those nearest and dearest to them (who are losing the care they have become used to). The whole world may suddenly appear to be conspiring to need their care most desperately. In my experience it is not enough, and often unhelpful, to challenge the compulsive caregiving and admonish the person to look after themself better. What is required is very detailed and diligent work to look at what happens when the client tries to receive something good and what gets in the way of them enjoying it. It may also be necessary to dissect what exactly happens to good things that the client has received, but then apparently unaccountably has lost, after a few minutes or a few days. Ultimately, I suspect that only real self-love may be able to shift this terrible defense that looks so good on the surface, is so encouraged by other people, and wreaks such havoc with a person's inner life and capacity for feeling joy.

I have previously alluded to the tangle of unpleasant experiences that has shaped Pearl's inability to receive good things. A reluctant mother, who was envious of the care she grudgingly gave her daughter, and felt herself to be deprived, with nothing to give to others, meant that Pearl was perhaps tolerated rather than loved and certainly didn't feel loved. Being given something she has longed for actually makes her anxious. She realizes that she is just waiting for the envious attack that will take it away again, leaving her intolerably bereft, shamed, and hurt. It becomes clear in the course of our work that this was indeed the pattern of her interactions with her mother, and Pearl still encounters it at times with her mother—who is now very elderly but still envious.

After a long time in therapy, Pearl gradually develops the idea that perhaps she just needs to find the love she needs elsewhere. We decide together that one way to do this will be for her to cultivate an awareness of just how many good things there might be in the world for her. We work hard to develop a certain openness for receiving such nourishing contact and emotional support that is given freely by people around her. After a while she says to me, "I'm surprised how often people do say nice things to me, and how many people really love me. I don't think I ever realized that properly." She sets up a self-help group of parents who struggle with teenage children, and she forms some very close and supportive friendships in this group. Over time, I observe that her ability to let go of the attempts to earn her mother's love decreases to the extent that her ability to accept love from others increases.

Early Emotional Neglect and Physical
Illness in Adulthood

In this section I will address two slightly different themes: the first is the impact that early emotional neglect has on the physical health of adults, and the second is a speculation about how early emotional neglect might predispose people to use *somatization*—that is, the expression of psychological distress as physical symptoms or physical disease—as a way of coping with the world.

The first topic, that of the ill-health sequelae of being an ignored child, makes for fairly worrying reading. Particularly traumatic birth experiences have been found to be strongly linked to conditions connected to impaired immune function: (1) chronic inflammatory conditions such as rheumatoid arthritis or inflammatory bowel disease and (2) conditions that are powerfully modulated by, or even arise from, chronic stress, such as diabetes, elevated blood pressure, and various allergic reactions (Herzog & Schmahl, 2018; Strathearn et al., 2001; Teicher et al., 2004). Chronic fatigue has also been linked to adverse childhood experiences including neglect (Goodwin et al., 2003; Heim et al., 2009). A recent meta-analysis comes to some very pessimistic conclusions indeed about the health prospects of people who were neglected in early childhood (Hughes et al., 2017).

There does not seem to be much difference between abuse and neglect as contributors to poor health in adulthood. What is consistently found is that the earlier neglect occurs, the more devastating its consequences are going to be. Conditions that involve weakened immune function seem common especially among those who were ignored children, which seems a further statement on the quality of their boundaries as well as on their ability to self-regulate.

One of the obvious causes of early neglect would be postnatal depression of the mother. The vast majority of studies of perinatal mental health issues are concerned with the mothers, not the children. The few studies that we have that investigate what happens to children of mothers with perinatal depression find effects on the cognitive and behavioral development of the children—who were followed up to age 4 years—but do not measure effects on physical health. Nevertheless, the authors of these studies seem confident that having a depressed mother constitutes a major adversity in childhood and quite likely a lifelong health risk (Maheu et al., 2010; Murray, 1992; Murray & Cooper, 1996).

I hope to have made the point by now that the autonomic nervous system (ANS) and, more broadly, the self-regulatory parts of the nervous system, are compromised in ignored children and don't cope well with stress, having only a narrow window of tolerance within which the person feels able to function at their best. We know that the immune system and the affect-regulatory parts of the nervous system talk to each other constantly and extensively through a multitude of signaling mechanisms (Pert, 1999). It is therefore easy to postulate that being ignored might affect a person's health by creating a constant background level of stress that in turn can be expected to affect their immune function.

The Center of the Developing Child at Harvard University has published an excellent brochure on foundations for lifelong health. In this brochure, the authors postulate the concept of toxic stress, explaining that "in contrast to positive or tolerable stress, toxic stress is defined as the excessive or prolonged activation of the physiologic stress response systems in the absence of the buffering protection afforded by stable, responsive relationships." They conclude that "the prevention of long-term, adverse consequences is best achieved by the buffering protection afforded by stable, responsive relationships that help children develop a sense of safety, thereby facilitating the restoration of their stress response systems to baseline" (Center of the Developing Child at Harvard University, 2010).

This concept of a balance between the load of stress, traumatic or otherwise, and the protective effect of being taken good care of seems to me to be very useful for therapists. It is not the amount or degree of childhood trauma suffered by an individual, but the balance between that and the positive experiences, the feelings of being loved and cared for, the available resources especially from nurturing contact, that determines how much we are going to suffer. A client might present with a horrific childhood history but with good interpersonal resources and might therefore be quite stable. On the other hand, another client may not know of many traumatic experiences in their childhood but may not have been well looked after and may not have a good network of supportive people currently—and this latter person may be more vulnerable than the former. Indeed, an argument could be made for saying that ignored children as a group fall into this latter category of people who may not have a horrendous history of terrible events but have not been given much or any protection against life's vicissitudes and are therefore going to be vulnerable to even minor life stresses.

As an image of how the human organism functions, we can conclude from these studies that feeling loved puts a protective buffer between us and difficult experiences, and that therefore we need love in order to be resilient (the attribute prized so much by today's corporate culture). This is an insight that has been intuitively available to many (see for example Rowling, 1997) but that has been slow to penetrate the more scientific world of acceptance of hard facts and aversion to "touchy-feely" notions of interpersonal contact. It may be worth saying that it is difficult to acquire this protective buffer in other ways than to be loved by another person, although if we have had the experience once, then therapy is quite good at helping us reestablish the connection to that experience and retain it in the future (see also Gerhardt, 2004).

I am now going to look at the tendency of ignored children to somatize. Somatization is a difficult concept that originally comes out of psychoanalytical thinking (see for example Alexander, 1950; Dethlefsen & Dahlke, 1993; Groddeck, 1949). The observation is rather old that some people seem to express their psychological distress in physical symptoms. In the early days of psychoanalysis, Freud's work on hysterical conversion offered a way of thinking about this, and a narrative developed that if a symptom was rooted in psychological distress, it was somehow not real—that is, it was not a physical illness requiring medical attention. To this day, we find many people with symptoms that have been labeled "psychological" who need to battle for the recognition of their symptoms as a legitimate physical condition with bodily causes. Slowly, it is becoming clear that a symptom can be perfectly real and still have its roots in, or at least be affected by, psychological distress (Bullington et al., 2003; Carroll, 2002b). Research on post-traumatic stress symptoms has done much to improve matters in this respect by showing that PTSD can present with many physical symptoms including chronic pain and conversion-like symptoms, which may respond to trauma therapy interventions (Kulich et al., 2000).

What is called somatization proper may be conceptualized as distress that is unbearable and overwhelms the organism's psychological self-regulatory mechanisms that have been acquired in early life, including the coping strategy of putting feelings into words as a way of holding them in mind. Names are very powerful containers, and being able to formulate a narrative for suffering makes much of it bearable and containable. If this is not available, we may speculate that a physical symptom results, as a way of putting the distress somewhere where it is no longer felt as life-threatening. We have to assume that this mechanism operates a long way out of conscious awareness and is untouched by any choices we may make. We can also assume that the origins of this way of containing distress can be placed in the time when the brain starts to elaborate bodily sensations into feelings, images, and words. I think it is sensible to think of somatization as a problem with symbolizing distress.

I hasten to add that in the short term, somatizing distress is a very successful coping strategy. In this respect it resembles dissociation (and a case can be made to regard somatization as a form of dissociation). It works tremendously well. Some forms of somatization lead to the secretion of endorphins in the bloodstream and thus provide a powerful and instant soothing of the whole organism. Even if this does not happen, a physical symptom represents a very strong container for suffering that would otherwise be unbearable. Moreover, physical illness provides a legitimate reason for the patient to be looked after and cared for; or it may provide a respectable narrative that the patient can understand; it often puts a boundary around the problem and limits it to a known amount of suffering for a limited amount of time. In addition, at least a young person can confidently look to a full recovery that will remove the problem altogether. The difficulties of somatization as a coping strategy arise more in the longer term. Indeed, it may not be until older age that people who somatize realize that there is a very high price to pay in terms of poor health and increased disability due to chronic conditions.

As discussed above, people are going to be prone to somatization if their psychological coping strategies (including interpersonal resources) are not well-developed and if at the same time they are subject to a large number of distressing experiences. We can see how this description fits ignored children, with the paucity of resources that result from developmental deficits. This is not to say that all ignored children somatize, but it seems to me that there is a tendency among them for shifting symptoms to the physical level.

There is a further factor that may well contribute to a propensity for people who have been ignored children to suffer from chronic conditions. This is the observation that ignored children learn early in life to ignore their own bodies and especially physical discomfort. Ignoring physical sensations often means that mild to moderate symptoms of illness get overlooked—until the illness becomes so severe that ignoring it is no longer possible. At this point illnesses can be more resistant to treatment and may persist for a long time.

There is often a slightly disembodied quality about ignored children and a sense that they don't entirely inhabit all of their bodies. Some ignored children are profoundly dissociated from their physical selves. Others feel ashamed of their bodies or of aspects of their physical being. Some also are frightened of the uncontrollable processes that happen in their bodies; this could be a generalized fear or more specific phobias such as fear of vomiting or a fear of particular illnesses like cancer or AIDS. All of these mind-body relationships mean that ignored children have a strong tendency to numb themselves to physical sensations.

Some ignored children are extremely terrified of physical symptoms and may ruminate about being seriously ill and about to die when they experience any change in their bodies. This makes for a very painful experience in life, where any body sensation is cause for alarm. In my experience, such fears often connect to early experiences of being abandoned and isolated in a frightening world. I think of them as flashbacks. Tragically, clients suffering from these fears tend to remain trapped in these flashbacks and are often unable to access help and support from others. Instead they may well look as if they are merely avoidant.

Olivia's health is always delicate, and she is always worried about it. At the same time, she struggles to get medical attention because she is so ashamed of being a needy and difficult patient. Debating with herself when a visit to her family physician is justified can take up a tremendous amount of her time and energy. I keep being struck by how difficult it is for her to actually feel her own body. When I ask her for a body sensation, she usually either deflects the question or says "it feels fine." As she suffers quite a lot from various joint pains, I suggest to her to try some complementary therapies. She chooses yoga first and quickly finds that she cannot do it without exacerbating her pains. Next she tries the Alexander technique. This produces some initial improvement, but she really dislikes it, and after a while I find out that she struggles with the "correct posture" demand that she feels is inherent in Alexander technique. Eventually she discovers the Feldenkrais movement technique, and this is an immediate success. It takes place in a group that she enjoys; that helps to keep her going regularly. The atmosphere of exploring how it feels is just what she likes, and the gentleness of the approach makes it pleasant and relaxing. Over time it produces a real change in her degree of embodiment.

All of these ways of relating to their bodies, typical for adults who were ignored children, represent variations of estrangement from the physical comfort that a happy and fulfilled life can offer. They form additional hardships that ignored children have to struggle with throughout their lives. Hardships can range from the mild discomfort of clumsy movements that require excessive strength; to severely painful chronic illnesses; or to bewildering and frightening, medically unexplained conditions. They are a part of the suffering that makes me feel so much compassion for ignored children.

CHAPTER 5

General Principles for Psychotherapy with Adults Who Were Ignored Children

Up to this point I have concentrated on understanding the experience of ignored children, including how this experience has come about, taking into account both conscious and unconscious elements. The question now is, how does this understanding translate into psychotherapy?

All therapists know that understanding is in itself therapeutic. Clients will feel safer, more accepted, and more seen by a therapist who understands what it is like to have similar experiences. They will feel this way even if they do not perceive consciously that their therapist understands them. This is true for all clients in psychotherapy. For ignored children it is often a tremendous relief to sit with a person who understands rather than judges, blames, or humiliates them through lack of understanding. If the therapist is able to communicate their understanding to the client, this adds a big chunk of therapeutic benefit to the situation. If the therapist can do this in such a way that a slow deepening of the client's own understanding results, another big chunk is added.

If understanding is all therapists offer to clients who were ignored children, the therapeutic process will be extremely slow. Both therapists and clients may experience sessions as tedious and hard work for little gain. As it turns out, many ignored children are very happy to go along with more directive therapists who negotiate an agenda and make active interventions. It takes away the burden of having to make it all happen by themselves. I have long been interested in learning the kinds of active interventions that can help make the therapeutic process of ignored children easier and less lengthy.

I will make suggestions both for facilitating attitudes on the part of the therapist and also for more active interventions, all aimed at improving the quality of psychotherapy for clients who were ignored children. I have divided these suggestions into two chapters. In this chapter I will address the points that are relevant for how therapists set up and conduct a therapeutic relationship with ignored children and the relational considerations that they need to keep in mind for this type of work. In Chapter 6, I will introduce specific interventions that I have found helpful.

I have further divided this chapter into my "seven major dos and don'ts" for psychotherapy with adults who were ignored children. Here is the list:

1. Create safety.
2. Don't challenge or confront.
3. Think in terms of deficits rather than conflicts.
4. Dose all interventions small enough to lead to an experience of success.
5. Keep in mind the client's shame including the shame of having to be in therapy.
6. Always remember that the client may not be able to express disagreement with you.
7. Be aware that good feelings may seem threatening to the client.

The rest of this chapter will be devoted to comments and explanations of these dos and don'ts. They arise out of my clinical experience and may need adapting by therapists who work in different ways that I do; but I have tried to distil the principles that can be applied by any psychotherapist.

Safety and Containment

Safety has to always be kept in mind. Safety may be the bottom line of life for ignored children, and without it they are left exposed to a world that one of my clients has described as "too full of wild dogs with sharp teeth"—a world filled with danger, humiliation, and failure. Even after several years of therapeutic work, the boundary that separates a safe therapeutic relationship from this frightening world can be extremely thin and fragile.

One of the really useful ways of building safety in a therapeutic relationship is the repair of a rupture in attachment. Unfortunately, this is also a major challenge for many ignored children who may form extremely insecure attachments. They may never have experienced even the possibility of repairing a relational rupture. We therefore have to regard rupture and repair as a high-risk strategy in the therapy with clients who were ignored children, and it may be better to think of alternatives. On a similar note, in my experience working through negative transference is a long way down the list of priorities in the therapy of ignored children.

In order to avoid catapulting the client into attachment ruptures prematurely, it is of crucial importance to establish and maintain a strong working alliance. Clients who were ignored children are well able to function on the level of the working alliance and, certainly in the early stages of a therapeutic process, to affirm the working alliance regularly will build a lot of safety for anxious clients. The working alliance in this way becomes the level at which rupture and repair can take place, rather than the transferential or developmentally needed relationship level (for my terminology of different levels of therapeutic relationship see Clarkson, 1995). I find this a more helpful strategy, on the whole, than attempting to attune so finely to the client that we avoid ruptures altogether. Most adults who were ignored children are very good at functioning on the level of a reasonable adult, and this means that they can maintain a good working alliance. This working alliance is often strong enough to hold minor ruptures and disagreements and misattunements.

What this means in practice is that if I notice that I have said something my client has found upsetting, I apologize for this and clarify that it was just a mistake on my behalf. This way I remain in the working alliance rather than encourage the client's thoughts and feelings about what they heard, which would be inviting a more transferential level. The downside of this maneuver is that I may lose some opportunities to explore the inner world of my client; the upside is that my client probably feels reassured by my willingness to own my mistakes and apologize and doesn't feel blamed for the rupture to our relationship.

If ruptures occur, as they are wont to do, it is important for ignored children to experience a therapist who does not put the onus for the repair on to the client. This would be adding to the burden of having to do everything for themselves that ignored children generally already suffer from. It will also repeat any blame and humiliation that ignored children are likely to have experienced in the past. In my experience, clients who were ignored children appreciate a therapist who is prepared to own their contribution to a rupture freely and to go the extra mile in repairing the relationship. I find that clients who were ignored children do well with a therapist who takes on more than their fair share of the work of building and maintaining a relationship, although I will try and attune this to the stage of the therapeutic process with each client, relying on the client to gradually take on more of this relational work.

I recommend for therapists to make sure they have a fairly wide repertoire for building safety, so that they can choose the best from a number of interventions. This recommendation applies to working with clients who were ignored children generally and not only to relational work. I find it helpful not to be attached to particular interventions but to be able to jettison an intervention that isn't working and try another one without much ado. I believe that this models a helpful way of being in the world to clients who tend to overrely on too few resources.

In working on safety, there should be two aims. (1) The client should become less dependent on their environment for safety and more in contact with what safety they have inside, and (2) The client should become able to create safety for themself. The two aims are similar and related. I consider them important and have found that particularly the latter can help build a stronger sense of self-agency in ignored children. It may be good to make these aims clear to the client, and to co-opt their collaboration. It may be of equal importance to state that an ignored child was not kept safe enough early in life and therefore has to rely on safety from another person for a while before being able to internalize this and build their own safety. It is probably helpful to think of the need for safety as another developmental deficit that needs to be filled before the person can develop independence. Safety in the therapeutic relationship should follow these aims, so that the client gradually becomes more able to co-create safety and decrease their dependency on the therapist's skills for safety-building.

Sometimes a lengthy period of work will be necessary until ignored children take their own need for safety seriously. Especially when the client has a very difficult relationship with their inner child, it is common for them to dismiss and disregard this child's need for safety. "She should just stop being a nuisance," or "I'm really fed up with how pathetic he is" are statements frequently heard. With these clients, I often spend quite a bit of time educating them about the physiological effects of anxiety or working with their inner child to improve their self-compassion. Regardless of whether clients are able to see the need for safety as legitimate or whether they try to deny, dismiss, or fight it, the therapist has to pay attention to it, because the need is always there and does not depend on the relationship the client happens to have with it.

Olivia often has great difficulties taking her need for safety seriously. It is clear that to her, feeling afraid of anything at all is shameful, and therefore she tries to ignore feelings of anxiety. "I look at other people and they all seem fine—I am the only one who is so flawed and pathetic," she says. This attitude is strengthened by the fact that she has spent a large part of her life successfully coping with constant high anxiety, so therefore it must be okay to ignore it. I try to explain my view that if she could live with less background anxiety, she would be much better in many ways and that reducing her anxiety necessitates taking it seriously and working on anxiety-management strategies. She is not able to follow my advice in this; rather she becomes more ashamed and withdraws from me. It is lucky that we have a good enough relationship that I notice the change in the quality of our contact. I say, "It looks like I said the wrong thing at some point—can you say what it was?" In response she can explain how ashamed she feels every time she thinks of getting anxious and how severely she takes herself to task for this weakness, and my suggesting she should be doing something different from what she is doing makes her feel more shame.

This little exchange, which is typical for our work, seems to contribute to slowly building a little relational safety. Olivia's tendency to ignore her anxiety reflects her own relationship with her anxious self, which is one of harsh criticism and generally feeling let down. Together we start to deliberately work on this internal relationship, creating a picture of her anxious inner child and working to understand where this child is coming from. At first, it is difficult for her to even visualize the anxious child, and she needs my reassurance that we can do this together. Gradually she begins to be able to see the anxious child and feel some empathy. As her attitude slowly changes over several years, the day finally comes when Olivia says, "Nowadays I am much better at spotting things that will make the Little One anxious, and I really want to protect her now."

Creating safety needs to be individualized and may be different for each individual. Feeling safe is a subjective experience that takes place in the context of the totality of the client's life experience, and we can never know all of that. Therefore, it is important for therapists not to expect that, just because they are intending to create safety, or because their textbook or their supervisor says that an intervention will create safety, this will necessarily be true for any individual client. We always have to check whether an intervention has indeed this result and be prepared to modify or jettison many strategies before finding the ones that work.

Having said that, I want to make some suggestions that are fairly likely to work. Here are a few of the therapeutic attitudes and interventions that can be expected to create safety for ignored children:

- The therapist needs to be warm but not invasive. The client should feel that they are welcome but that the therapist isn't making any demands on them. This may be a challenge to therapists who like to be seen as warm and caring. Building a relationship with an ignored child can be like taming a feral or wild animal—it takes patience and a lot of readiness to be run away from and come back to. It is important not to take clients' rejections of a therapist's attempt to make contact personally. Instead therapists need to understand that ignored children will often reject such overtures in order to protect themselves from disappointment, exploitation, or invasion. It can be a challenge to some therapists to continue to show warmth to somebody who does not return warmth.

- Silence is anxiety-provoking and can be experienced as a reenactment of a withdrawn or absent caregiver. Many therapists think it respectful to wait for the client to start the session. I recommend changing this habit for ignored children and just saying something very neutral and inviting. My experience suggests that faced with a silent person, many ignored children are left at the mercy of their punitive introjects and will very rapidly fall prey to harsh and abusive internal self-talk, or even drop into distressing flashbacks, unless they are reliably prevented from this by a friendly and supportive therapist who makes just enough contact to hold them in a more resourced self-state.

- I have learned to pay attention to the physical environment of the therapy. Basic aspects like the distance between myself and the client and the orientation of our chairs to not directly face each other but stand at a slight angle, as well as the choice of clients either to be near the door (for a fast getaway) or to keep an eye on the door (to monitor for intrusions) are worth keeping in mind and at times modifying according to client's perceived anxiety. I will not, of course, compromise my own safety and comfort, but when it doesn't matter to me, I will adjust to the wishes of my clients. Some of my clients will sit with a cushion on their lap to protect the vulnerable front of their bodies, and others find different ways of making sessions more comfortable and safer. Having soft materials like blankets and cushions in the room has many therapeutic applications and always seems a good idea. For many adults who were ignored children, being looked at feels exposing and difficult, and it may be good for the therapist to teach themselves not to look directly at the client much of the time and also to keep the gaze soft.

• Ignored children tend to have a vast longing for someone to be in charge, for a benign authority figure. After all, this is what they missed in their early life. Many therapists are taught to regard a therapeutic relationship as a relationship of equals, but for ignored children it may be necessary to modify this idea. It is especially important to avoid creating a relationship in which the client feels they need to look after the therapist. On the other hand, it is also a tremendous opportunity for the therapist to use their authority in order to direct the therapeutic process. If we look at the origin of the word "authority," its literal meaning is "the power to grow things." A benevolent therapist who knows where to start the process of therapy and which directions to pursue is the kind of parental figure that many ignored children need in order to heal and grow. If clients who were ignored children feel that the therapist knows what needs to happen for them to get better, they are more likely to trust their therapist and feel safe with them. If on the other hand they see the therapist attempting to create a more equal relationship, they may feel out of their depth and faced with unmanageable demands, and they may become anxious or resort to compulsive caregiving.

- It may create further safety if the therapist is able to work in a very transparent way. Some ignored children may not particularly want to know what the therapist is aiming for and prefer for the process to be a bit magical, but others will greatly appreciate the added sense of control that they get from a therapist who can explain what they are doing and why. Therapists need to consider the needs of each client in this respect and be able to adopt either style of working. In turn, working in a very transparent manner will strengthen the working alliance and make the therapy far less fatiguing and easier for the therapist.

Avoiding Challenges and Confrontations

The second major don't of therapy for ignored children is challenges or confrontations. There are several reasons that challenges are unlikely to benefit the therapy of ignored children and may destroy a lot of trust and motivation. One reason is the toxic and indigestible shame that most ignored children feel. It creates a state of mind in which the person is forever examining all their thoughts and behaviors for anything that may be at fault or that could be attacked. This means that if the therapist challenges a thought, feeling, or action of the client, the client will likely already have thought of the challenge and know they cannot meet it. Most of us know that it is most annoying and humiliating to be criticized for something that we already feel bad about! It is therefore to be expected that such a challenge will lead to further shame. Alternatively, if the client has not thought of the challenge, they will feel caught out and embarrassed precisely because of this.

It is also important to remember that clients who were ignored children tend to implode in shame, rather than to get angry or ward the shame off in some other way. It may therefore not be obvious to the therapist that the client feels shamed.

A second reason is the desperately insecure attachment that many ignored children form to their therapist. It is important to remember that ignored children will almost certainly jump to the conclusion that the therapist is angry and therefore about to reject them. Even a mild challenge may well signal to an ignored child that they are unacceptable and will be cast into outer darkness. The fear that is likely to result from this will forestall any therapeutic benefit. This fear will also likely swamp any anger that might be present (and that the therapist who challenges might want to elicit), so that the client in all honesty cannot feel it.

There is a third reason to avoid challenges: ignored children live constantly with emotions that are so strong they can barely be coped with. I see the wish of ignored children to keep life on an even keel and avoid excitement as a legitimate attempt to make things more manageable for themselves. Ignored children do better when therapists respect this wish and help them create more constancy and safety. Challenges risk being too much for the client to integrate and can thus easily be re-traumatizing. Decisions to give the client's emotional muscle some exercise need to be carefully considered by any therapist wishing to challenge their client. I will comment on this further in the section on Dosing Down.

It is one of the major countertransference pitfalls with clients who were ignored children for a therapist to challenge their client without quite realizing that the client is not in a position to benefit from such a challenge. The danger here is that the therapist merely reenacts the client's habitual transference of being shamed, blamed, and bullied. Like all reenactments this can be turned to therapeutic benefit but requires a therapist who is skilled at working in this particular way.

Clients who were ignored children present with anxieties that are not the result of unconscious conflicts, as is a typical assumption in classical psychodynamic psychotherapy. This means that many of the interventions of classical psychotherapy, such as interpreting or confronting, will not be therapeutically effective. This caveat is also part of the consideration of thinking about deficit rather than conflict and constitutes a further reason not to challenge or confront.

Many therapists will ask what alternative interventions I suggest. My approach is that the therapist needs to do more work reflecting on the meaning that the client's attitude or behavior that they are wanting to challenge is likely to have for the client, at as much depth of which they are capable. It may be possible to do that in the moment, or the therapist may access supervision for the purpose. In my experience, it is usually possible to reframe a challenge in such a way that it turns into support and opens more inner space for the client. In relational terms, this means that the therapist needs to shoulder more of the burden of the work done in the relationship.

The following may illustrate just how this kind of work can look:

One day I come up against Pearl's inability to set boundaries toward other people's demands. This has happened often, and many times I have tried to address her fear of others' displeasure and feeling abandoned. I have never felt that I was doing anything useful by this type of intervention, so this time instead of going down the well-trodden path, I sit back and think how I would formulate Pearl's inability to say no to others. If there were a good reason for it, what could it be? I know about her fear of being rejected, but is that really the whole story? As I sit with these questions, it occurs to me that her refusal to look after herself feels almost as though there is a stronger loyalty involved with which she has to keep faith. I decide to risk being wrong, and say, "It almost feels as though you made a decision very early on in your life that you would never abandon other people as you have been abandoned." She looks stricken and then acknowledges that this is exactly it, that this is the part of herself that she has desperately clung to all the time. In the following sessions I can then support this decision and help her negotiate a more lenient interpretation, so that looking after herself finds a little space in her life as well. Over a period of time, having shared with me what is really happening inside her creates a softening in Pearl. Eventually it leads to a relaxing of her dilemma where looking after herself would make it impossible to look after others, and she gradually arrives at a position where she can do a bit of both. Understanding and naming her passionate clinging to her ability to do better than her mother proves to be a turning point in her therapeutic process.

I hope this shows the way I may work to get out of stalemates created by inappropriate challenges. I use all that I know about the client and all the information I access from my physical and emotional resonance with them, in order to build a model of how they function and what their main motivations are, both conscious and unconscious. Then the task is to feed these motivations back to the client in a form that they can feel seen and supported by. This works best if I have established a therapeutic relationship in which it is clear to the client that I am curious about how accurate or inaccurate my speculations are, and I am looking to them to provide me with this feedback. I would of course want to avoid getting it wrong and manipulating them into believing something about their own inner life that isn't actually true, so I have to look out for signs of that—and sometimes I just have to trust that they will find a way to let me know, even in a very roundabout manner.

Another possibility would be to anticipate the shame of a client when confronted with a perceived weakness of his and making this part of my intervention, as follows:

> Mortimer keeps telling me how he dislikes being in company and left to his own devices would always choose just to sit at home by himself. I know that he has often been told he is odd, weak, defective, or cowardly for this attitude. So I decide not to add my voice to those many voices that are already in his head but say something like: "I can see that this is very difficult for you. If you have already been told off so many times, there must be a lot of anger in you, and that will of course feed the fear of being in company with others and also the shame about it. It's bound to be a real uphill struggle!" His response to this is a slightly rueful smile, and he starts to tell me about the anger. The defensiveness in his voice is now gone, and we can both breathe more easily in the space around the subject.

A question that may be asked at this point is how to recognize whether by avoiding challenges the therapist is colluding with a malignant regression in the client. There is no simple answer to this. Therapists who work with regressed self-states ("inner child work") probably all know that there is no certain way of checking whether the process is leading to therapeutic gain in the longer term or whether the client just gets stuck and cannot develop further. As a rule of thumb, we can look at the client's functioning over a period of weeks and months and see whether they are getting better or worse and whether we are therefore building new resources or re-traumatizing the client by maintaining a fragmentation. I may add that confronting the client seems unlikely to be a therapeutically useful way out of this dilemma.

The following section will provide some more insight into why challenges need to be avoided or at least crafted very carefully and skillfully with clients who were ignored children.

Deficit Orientation

One of the most salient traits of ignored children is the presence of developmental deficits. I find that on the whole psychotherapy has struggled to develop strategies for working with such deficits. Working to fill in what is lacking is crucial to the work with clients who were ignored children. I have an image of the mind of ignored children full of holes, held together with a fine net of resources that have to take the whole strain of dealing with life's stresses and vicissitudes. This image keeps reminding me of just how few resources most ignored children have.

It is my observation that under favorable conditions many deficits will spontaneously fill up, but in adults who were ignored children and are still affected by that experience these favorable conditions are rarely present. Moreover, the paucity of resources makes these clients vulnerable to being set back by relatively minor disruptions to their lives. At the same time, we can derive a possible direction for the therapy from this idea: if we manage to provide favorable conditions, deficits may fill up spontaneously. This is rather like the "Reprocessing" stage of EMDR, which tends to happen spontaneously when the desensitization is completed.

Having said that, it still remains a major therapeutic challenge to work with clients who have missed out on many developmental steps, especially early in life. Therapists need to create a space of acceptance and gentle nurturing that invites clients to relax and feel good. We need to think about how to awaken our clients' creativity and their capacity for curiosity and learning. We need to learn to spot a small vestige of a resource and work to help it grow and spread. We need to be undeterred by the client's attempts to cling to old and tried resources and avoid learning new ones. We need to be prepared to meet with some very ingenious maneuvers by our clients to avoid changing, and to spend time unraveling these maneuvers to the point where they can be understood and appreciated and hopefully relax their stranglehold.

Creative imagination seems to play a pivotal role in therapy that aims to fill in deficits. Images, dreams, and visions build soul and are some of the most powerful mental and spiritual resources for human beings. If clients can imagine something, this image is a seed that can grow into a real experience or a new skill. Imagination tends to open the mind and do so in a pleasurable manner that will not trigger the usual reflex responses of avoidance out of fear. Most ignored children can readily visualize images, and it is often worthwhile to capitalize on this strength.

Another way of filling in deficits is the reparative, or developmentally needed, relationship that therapists can build with ignored children (Clarkson, 1995). It seems likely that this will always happen to an extent, but therapists may be more or less comfortable with the idea. Ignored children may fall in love with their therapists and thus form a powerful attachment relationship. If the therapist can make space for this feeling in the therapy room in a safe and appropriate way, the therapy may be very reparative and change a life for the better. This is by no means necessary for good therapy, and many interventions can help to create experiences of beneficial interpersonal contact that are healing and at the same time expand the mind.

Let me bring in Norman here. After some months of working with him he discloses that he has fallen in love with me. I respond welcoming his feelings, emphasizing that loving feelings are a sign that he is involved in the process and really wants to get better—rather like a commitment that he has made to himself. His loving feelings are a way into the aliveness that he has hitherto missed in himself and the hope that such feelings can heal not just the person who receives them but also the person who is having them in the first place. In passing, I also state that we will not be having a sexual relationship. He accepts this boundary without much comment.

In the following weeks, I am careful to give him enough space to talk about how he feels toward me. I expect longing and at the same time embarrassment, humiliation, frustration, anger, and grief, and perhaps more: after all, he is bound to feel rejected by me, so I am prepared for the feelings that should go with this situation. He doesn't voice any of that except, very cautiously, longing. I ask whether there are any other feelings. He says no, and after some weeks explains that if he feels anything "negative," he risks losing what little he has. He cannot quite understand how anybody who is in love could possibly allow such negative feelings—that just seems crazy to him. I feel troubled at being shown what his inner world looks like. The sense that he expects so much pain no matter what he says in this situation is almost suffocating and distressing to be with.

This continues for months. At times I feel deep shame for my inability to love him as he deserves to be loved. All I am able to do during these months is reiterate what he can have: I am here, I am fond of him, we make good contact, he feels understood and seen. I have tremendous doubts about the therapy as a whole. Every week I expect Norman to terminate the sessions. Part of me wishes him to do so for his own protection. I think it entirely possible that the relationship is abusive and just re-traumatizing him, and that he cannot integrate what is happening. After some months,

I have a long conversation with my supervisor and understand that these thoughts are part of my countertransference: my shame and helpless worry are the closest to love that he is able to elicit in such an insecure attachment relationship.

I feel encouraged to link more firmly with the reflective part of him that can see what is happening and what might be a way out. Eventually he creates a connection between what is happening now and his childhood, and with that he can start to grieve for how awful his situation was then and how awful it is now. Gradually he becomes more able to think deeply about his childhood and how he himself can understand it. From that time on, he begins to integrate feelings and thoughts more easily and learns to allow himself actually to have what there is in the sessions for him: a deep affection that we have for each other, the easy contact and understanding, and the messages from me that he is a worthwhile human being.

In this context a word should be said about the difference between malignant regression and therapeutically productive regression, which (as my example shows) can be a difficult distinction to make. Many practitioners seem to agree that the decisive factor is integration. If a client can integrate a *reparative experience* into the stream of their autobiographical self, so that they are left more complete, more resourced, and more able to grow and transform, then the experience has had a good effect. If on the other hand the experience remains separate or even becomes a dreamed-of paradise lost that will hijack all the client's vital energy in an effort to return to it, then it is likely that the therapy will not lead to a good outcome; rather, it will have strengthened a traumatized fragment of the client that is unable to exert a beneficial effect on the whole personality but instead acts more like an addiction to an unhealthy substance. Therapists should be able to reflect on their own work in a dispassionate and mature way in order to spot these malignant processes and be able to change the direction of the therapy if necessary.

Dosing Down

It is part of healthy self-regulation to rise to challenges. If we successfully deal with them, they leave us with a sense of achievement that will become the foundation for self-confidence and the motivation and courage to tackle future challenges. It seems likely that praise or appreciation from authority figures will enhance the good experience of achievement and help to create more confidence.

It is trivial to say that the size of a challenge should always be in proportion to the resources for meeting it that the client has. Everybody would agree to this when we talk about the education of children. However, clients who were ignored children have typically had far too many experiences of trying to cope with challenges that were way beyond them, followed by the humiliation and shame associated with failing at the task. They may have had to cope with far too much far too soon as children, and therefore challenges may be experienced as threatening situations to be avoided at all costs. This creates a vicious cycle that stops ignored children from becoming able to trust their own abilities. Ignored children typically do not even try to tackle challenges, and if they do, they quickly give up.

Many ignored children learn to cope with challenges as they grow up, by making themselves tackle them in order to avoid being disabled by their fear and avoidance. They will probably put immense amounts of effort into being well prepared and making sure they have all possible skills for succeeding. This almost inevitably becomes a drain on their vitality and may lead to burnout. Moreover, I often observe that such effortful ways of meeting challenges don't seem to build much confidence, possibly because they come at such a high price; it seems to me a worthwhile therapeutic endeavor to attempt to make life a little easier in this respect.

The best way of getting around this obstacle is probably to decrease the sizes of the challenges. We can imagine muscles that have never developed much and remain weak. If we try to make such muscles work hard, they will quickly become overwhelmed by fatigue or even pain and give up. If we continue to try to make them work hard, the result will just be more fatigue and pain. If we want to develop the strength in such muscles, we have to give them just the right amount of work to do, small enough so that they can manage. When we get this dose just right, there will be a sensation of achievement in the muscles, a good feeling that builds confidence. Then the muscles can gradually build up their strength. The same applies to motivational muscle. Faced with clients whose natural response to a challenge is a resigned turning away or fearful avoidance, we need to create smaller challenges, or *dose down*.

Clients who were ignored children have, in addition, a tendency to perceive challenges where others might not. Many compare themselves relentlessly to more successful people and those who can access more support. The internal persecution the ignored children suffer will inevitably point out to them how substandard they are in every way. The shame engendered by these thoughts will stop many clients from communicating them to their therapist. It is best to learn to spot the subtle signs indicating that the client feels overwhelmed with a task. Then the therapist can backpedal and make the task smaller. I also find that it is a good idea to tell clients that this is what I am doing. They can then understand why I will not support their tendency to seek heroic challenges that are beyond them in an effort to shortcut a long and tedious process.

The following example may show how this could look in practice:

> Mortimer shows the typical inattention to how big a challenge anything represents for him as he contemplates looking for a new job. He is full of fear of what a terrible situation he will put himself in if he gives up his current job and moves from the familiar environment to a new and unfamiliar one.
>
> I point out to him that it would be therapeutically valuable if he could manage to break the task down into more manageable chunks. I remind him of the earlier piece of work for which we found ways to stack up the odds of a challenge in his favor and that this worked. After some argument, he agrees, and together we create a list of steps including the possibility of changing jobs gradually by reducing the number of hours he works in his old job in line with increasing the number of hours in the new job. It takes some time, but 6 months later he has managed to change to a new job without experiencing major episodes of panic or feeling defeated most of the time. He is pleased with the result, and when we finish therapy, he will name the ability to "make lists" as one of his more memorable gains from therapy.

Shame in the Therapeutic Relationship

One of the most disheartening realizations for therapists can be that for clients who were ignored children there is often virtually no space between therapy and humiliation. Having to be in therapy is humiliating, and so is having to submit to the authority of a therapist and having to reflect on one's own shortcomings for hour after hour. The very fact of being in therapy goes counter to the habitual avoidance of ignored children and pushes them into their most shameful places.

Imagine not being shown how to manage life and having to teach yourself how to be a proper person while always suspecting that you are not getting it quite right. This kind of shame-filled existence becomes torture when you see a therapist whose job it is—so you assume—to show you all the ways in which you should have been doing things better all along. I have met with many ignored children who lived in exactly such an inner world and who had to endure a massive amount of humiliation in order even to turn up for therapy sessions.

Such shame can contaminate the whole therapy, and clients will need a powerful motivation to continue the process. In order to provide such motivation quickly after the start of therapy, it is desirable for the therapist to be a good enough relational match for the client to feel seen and understood. It is also beneficial if the therapist can keep the emotional climate of sessions light and matter-of-fact (without appearing to make light of the client's suffering), as this may help make the experience bearable for the client. Experiences of shared laughter and humor can also be beneficial, as long as they don't make fun of something about which the client feels ashamed.

Any intervention that can diminish shame will be good to make. The first, and perhaps most important, is to name shame, adding that it is an ordinary part of the human condition. The more normal shame looks and sounds to the client, the easier it will be to process. It is also usually helpful if the therapist can model a fairly relaxed relationship with their own shame and embarrassment.

The point has been made that the shame of ignored children can be assumed to be a sign of the "identification with the aggressor" they suffer from (Schimmenti, 2012). In other words, the shame results from the inability of an ignored child to bear their experience of being unwanted, unacceptable, or disgusting. In order to escape it, the child identifies with the experience of the parent—who may be making judgments about the failings of the child in order to justify their own neglectful actions. It is often a long and hard therapeutic process to undo this identification. In this situation, we are therefore faced with a client who is split in two parts: the introjected caregiver who is judgmental and shaming, and the inner child who is ashamed. Ultimately the way out of this split will include both to help protect the shamed child and also to separate from the shaming introject. When clients disclose shameful secrets to me, I am careful to show some empathy while also mirroring back that they are feeling embarrassed and humiliated and that I think well of them for having disclosed the secret so that it can lose some of its toxicity. How exactly I balance my interventions will depend on how I perceive the relationship between the shamed child and the shaming introject. If it seems safe to support the shamed child without attacking the parental introject I will do that; if the parental introject is also in need of some support, or if the identification of my client with the parental introject is still very powerful, then I will give a more neutral response.

I have already written about Olivia's shame because she has to keep me at bay despite her own wish for closer connection with other people. The first time she discloses this to me I emphasize my conviction that there is a good reason for her inability to allow more closeness, and I state my willingness to work with her on finding out what that might be. This produces some relief, and we can explore the thoughts and feelings that produce shame. After a little further work, she realizes that she is caught on the horns of a dilemma between the shame connected to her inability to get close to others, and the shame of needing others rather than being independent. I ask her to imagine having these two parcels of shame in either hand and getting a sense of which weighs more heavily. She gets a clear sense that the shame of needing others is heavier. We further find that it is closely allied to the shame of being abandoned by her genetic mother.

Between these many parcels of shame, I cannot see how to intervene without adding shame to at least one of them. Mindful of her statement about how weighty the different parcels are, I address the shame of being unable to change early in therapy, and the shame about being given away by her birth mother much later. There is some risk here for me: My own shame around intervening too forcefully is likely to get triggered when we talk about what prevents her from changing, and I have to sit with my resulting feelings of being an insensitive and persecutory therapist.

We start to work on how ashamed she feels of being abandoned by her mother when we talk about how she relates to the baby that she once was, and how she tends to heap more shame on this baby in an effort to protect the more adult part of herself from being totally crippled by that shame. By this stage, we have established a good understanding of how to be with shame between the two of us, and it is much easier to access these deeper layers of shame. All my interventions are aimed at communicating my understanding of the difficult knots of shame that have permeated Olivia's whole existence.

I feel it important to frame my clients' shame as part of their past experience—a traumatic introject resulting from their early experience of being neglected or of a specific trauma. This makes it possible to talk about it with a little more distance. It also makes it clear that I think they are not shameful in any way without making them ashamed of being so full of shame. Once shame has been contextualized in this way as part of an earlier experience, we can then start to disentangle the strands of it and see the shame that may not be theirs, the shame that may be a normal part of life and can be shrugged off, and the shame that may lead us still further into the story of their early experiences. In the course of such lengthy work, most clients become much more able to digest shame and much less disabled by it.

Work with Very Insecurely Attached Clients Who Cannot Say No

I have found that ignored children who form very fragile bonds of attachment are extremely difficult to read. We can understand this from the finding that in an early attachment relationship, when the caregiver is not attuning to the baby, the baby will reverse the dynamic and attune to the caregiver. When this happens, it is very easy for the baby to be overfocused on the emotional life of the caregiver to the point that the baby cannot access their own feelings; their facial expression and body language will mirror the other person rather than express their own feelings. This way of being can be reactivated in adulthood if the person is in a relationship that seems very precarious. It is as though they are clinging so desperately to the little contact they have that the act of letting go for long enough to find out how they feel in themselves is unthinkably dangerous. It is dangerous because it threatens to catapult them into the void of total isolation—a scenario that has been called every human being's worst terror.

It is also important to be aware that for insecurely attached clients, the attachment will always be prioritized over self-expression. They have no choice about this—it is an automatism. This means that with the best will in the world, such clients may not be able to let the therapist know how they are receiving the therapy, because their need to placate the therapist will be too powerful. In my experience it is a very important part of working relationally that we inquire into the subject of what happens to our interventions in the inner world of the client and how this develops between sessions. This inquiry is difficult to conduct with ignored children. It may leave therapists guided by their own good intentions only and thus put clients at risk from being imposed upon or, in a reenactment of the original injury, ignored at a deeper level. Therapists may see clients who seem to be extremely satisfied with the therapy, because these clients do not have a choice but, in a reflex response, act to keep the therapist happy and themselves safe.

One of the ways out of this difficulty is to observe clients closely, especially over long periods of time. I want to know particularly whether the client can make use of the sessions to build new resources or if they somehow dismantle the gain from sessions afterwards. If a client keeps forgetting what we have talked about, or if I feel they are dismissing the therapy as unimportant, or if they seem to argue with a session afterward to the point that they reject it, then I will assume that there is a discrepancy between what they say when in my presence and what they think when they are not in my office. Other ways of preventing such cul-de-sacs include paying more attention to the client's nonverbal expressions and behavior than to what they say, paying attention to the quality of the contact, and offering the client the possibility of disagreeing with the therapist in a way that doesn't threaten the relationship. The latter strategy will only work when the therapeutic relationship has already developed a fair amount of relational safety.

Here is an example of how I might address Norman's discomfort with a casual comment of mine about politics that makes him realize that his political perspective is very different from mine.

He is not able to voice his discomfort and becomes very silent for several sessions. My questions get no useful answers, and this very fact tells me that something is not right between us and that Norman cannot tell me. Eventually I say, "It seems to me that you are rather distant these days. I wonder if I have said something that has offended you, although I imagine you might not want to say that because it might make matters worse. I can imagine that when I say offensive things, I deprive you of the comfort of your loving feelings, and that is very painful for you." He agrees that he has had difficult feelings about me without giving me much detail. We then have a little conversation about how we might be able to restore the good feeling that is usually in the room between us. I deliberately frame the problem as "difference" rather than as "conflict." Once he feels confident that I would want to help him restore his loving feelings and that we can probably find a way together, he is able to say in a fairly matter-of-fact way that he disagrees with my political views and struggles to work out what this might mean. This opens the space for a further exploration of how we can be with this difference and what it means for our relationship and gradually brings us back into good contact with each other again. The whole cycle takes several sessions but the therapeutic gain for Norman is considerable, giving him an experience of a relationship that doesn't depend on an ability to be merged with an idealized other, but that trusts the relational bond and can allow for difference.

In order to arrive at a more realistic assessment of a therapeutic process, I also rely on the little reenactments that I get pulled into with my clients to inform me that I am caught in a process that isn't quite as straightforward as it appears on the surface. Again, this requires work on my part and a good internal and external supervisor. And, as is typical in working with ignored children, I need all my ability for compassionate understanding.

It seems to me that in the last 20 years or so, the psychotherapy profession as a whole has had to learn just how unequal the relationship between therapist and client generally is. It has also had to learn that clients who are insecurely attached form particularly asymmetric relationships and are particularly vulnerable to misuses of power. This development may have taken place because of the more fragile ego structures of contemporary therapy clients. It may also be due to the greater skill of therapists who have developed a broad range of styles for working in an unequal relationship. Of course societal developments in the area of intersectionality have contributed to sharpening the alertness of therapists to power issues. It seems clear to me that the potential for all sorts of misuses of power in therapeutic relationships with clients who were ignored children is great, especially when therapists feel really uncomfortable acknowledging the power differential between themselves and their clients. I believe that part of becoming a good psychotherapist is to work through the relationship we ourselves have with power, for good and for ill.

When Feeling Good Becomes Threatening

Ignored children are somewhat prone to what has been called the *negative therapeutic reaction*, the observation that when therapeutic gain has been made, the client responds to this by getting worse. This may mean that the client becomes more anxious or that they develop anxiety about an area of their lives that has not previously caused them much concern.

I have explored several such responses from clients and come across several possible underlying scenarios. I have not encountered such a reaction that was the result of malicious or vengeful intent on the part of the client toward me or that was exclusively the result of some secondary gain that the client experienced from their suffering. I am therefore not much of a believer in the secondary gain hypothesis and would see it as a factor of subordinate importance in stabilizing a neurotic behavior or trait. On the other hand, I have often encountered clients who were ignored children whose neurotic traits are stabilized by terror of what could happen when they are given up. In the following I will outline the possible scenarios that I have met with that may account for the threat in feeling good that some ignored children experience. I do not claim that this list is complete but intend it as a suggestion. Other clinicians will no doubt find other dynamics at work.

One possibility is for the client to come from an environment of poverty, where there is great need combined with a scarcity of resources, resulting in a pervasive feeling of "there is not enough good to go around." This may be a material reality, or it may relate to more interpersonal good things such as attention, love, and support. In both cases the typical scenario is that too many people compete for too few resources, and this can imply that if one person gets something good, somebody else goes short; in other words, they are taking it away from somebody else. There may also be a sense that the person is physically too weak to fight for their own fair share, rather like the weakest of a large litter of kittens. For ignored children, who typically live with an imperative of privileging others over themselves in order to create a little safety, the feeling that they are taking something good away from somebody else can create an unbearable sense of threat. In the conscious awareness of the person this can then take the shape of a mindset of "I am tough, I can take deprivation or abuse better than others" or "It doesn't matter if I get hurt as long as others are happy." Many people with this type of belief do not present for psychotherapy until an illness or old age has led to the breakdown of this grandi-ose defense.

> The belief that anything good she has for herself is taken away from somebody else and means she is a selfish person is a constant companion for Pearl. Countless times she has been told, and understood—or so she assures me—that there is enough good in the world for everybody and she can have as much as she needs without being selfish or antisocial. Still, she herself tells me that "this seems to be a case where my thoughts don't have much influence over my feelings at all, and the feelings of being selfish and bad are just much stronger." Clearly there are some powerful beliefs there that she dare not discard because they might still be true. Over a period of time I work with her on the topic of selfishness and on the question of just how unbearable the feelings are. Feeling selfish or bad is unbearable for her, and a little deprivation is a small price to pay for avoiding such terrible feelings. She would be so anxious! Over time, she is willing to gamble on the anxiety decreasing in time as she braves the dreaded label and becomes a selfish person. Once she has managed to do that, there is even a part of her that starts to enjoy being selfish.

Another possibility is that the client has grown up with envious people. We can think of two possible forms of envy. One seeks to spoil and destroy anything good that another person has. The other seeks to ensure that the envious person gets the same good thing. The first of these two forms is a very destructive emotion. Between parents and their children this may take the form of, "I didn't have it easy and don't see why you should have it better," or it may be, "Don't think you're something special!" Between siblings the latter form is common, or there may be real rage toward a perceived preference given to the sibling that ends up destroying the good in the name of fairness. Whichever it is, children who grow up in an atmosphere where envious attacks are frequent may well end up not daring to have anything good. Worse, in an effort to preempt the shame and destruction visited upon them by other people's envy, they may attack and destroy their own achievements and resources. We can understand this both as an identification with the perpetrator and as an effort to forestall envious attacks. If you have a family that will not let you have anything good, you may carry out your own destruction because it actually doesn't hurt quite as much; you may also be caught up in forever hoping that you can attain a level of perfection that makes the good indestructible. In order to maintain this hope, you will have to test the good very hard in order to find any remaining weak spots. I find that this type of dynamic is often deeply buried, not easily accessible in therapy, and not easy to change. The only real winning strategy for people who have grown up in envious environments is to have what good they can despite their envious detractors. This requires enormous stamina and internal emotional support.

A similar scenario is present in many who have grown up and lived with the internalized persecution that they attract because of their membership of a section of society that is discriminated against (women, gender and sexual orientation minorities, ethnic minorities, etc.). Such internalized persecution functions in a very similar way and makes having anything good dangerous. It may also contribute to the avoidance of being "seen" that is experienced as being exposed by many who have been ignored children.

Finally, I have found in many ignored children a history of early loss of a good attachment. For these individuals, to lose something good is so traumatic and so dreaded that every gain of something good comes with a vast burden of fear lest it be lost again. Many of these persons have the conscious belief that "every time I start to enjoy myself, something terrible happens." This could be dismissed as mere superstition, but I find it more fruitful to assume that it is an actual memory or a chain of memories and work with it as such.

Sometimes more than one of these histories is present and results in a tighter knot of apparent resistance to getting better that requires more lengthy work to unravel. It is my experience that, once understood, these types of dynamics can slowly and gradually improve and need not cripple clients forever.

After many months of working, Mortimer gradually allows himself to fully experience the horror of the inescapable prison that forms his inner world. With more clarity and more ability to put words to his feelings comes more insight into how he was really treated by his very ambitious parents. Particularly his mother, who was depressed for some of his childhood, emerges as frequently unkind and destructive in her treatment of him. It takes a long time, and involves a lot of building his understanding of what life was like for his mother, to shift his tendency to savage himself and allow himself a little more success. He continues to feel that he does not deserve this. One day he suddenly says, "It's weird—part of me is very clear that I deserve the same as anybody else. But there is always this little voice inside that says you're nothing, you deserve nothing. As if that wasn't quite me." I ask whose the voice might be. "I suppose my mother's—she was usually my fiercest critic and taught me always to look for flaws. Now I can't imagine not doing that all the time and risking overlooking something that could be attacked." I pick up the fear of being attacked and ask how he thinks his more contemporary self might respond to this. At first he remains in the past and repeats how frightened he is of criticism. Then I remind him of a recent event when he experienced some criticism at work and actually was able to stand his ground and calmly explain why he had done the thing that got criticized. This helps him to see that his contemporary self has a host of resources to cope with attacks that his child self never had. His fear of attacks and criticism starts to diminish after that session.

Potential impediments to working through this very challenging issue include that therapists may start blaming their clients for "not wanting to get better." Therapists may also have powerfully hostile feelings toward a client who defies or thwarts their good intentions. Worst of all, there may well grow to be powerful collusions between clients and therapists who dislike, blame, and possibly bully the inner child who cannot process their experience of being ignored, rejected, and abandoned. Such a joint attack by therapist and client's superego will successfully stall any therapeutic process. The remedy is good supervision and a willingness on the part of the therapist to go deeper in their understanding until they unearth the motivation that truly represents the best the client was able to do in a difficult situation. The assumption that this motivation exists has never yet let me down.

It is common in clinical practice of psychotherapy to find clients who have learned to hate or despise their own young self. Clients who were ignored children are perhaps more prone than others to doing this, because they are so identified with a persecutor who may be hard to recognize as such and from whom it may be particularly difficult to separate. These clients can be seen as their own worst enemies and need to repair their relationship with their own child self, at least to a degree, before being able to benefit from therapy. Interventions using EMDR to help speed up this process are worth trying out (see for example Knight, 2008), as are two-chair type techniques (Perls, Hefferline & Goodman, 1951). I see this kind of identification with the aggressor as part of a traumatic early scenario. Its repair is part of the work of reassembling the integrity of the self. My favorite way of reframing it is to talk about clients' loyalty to their parents, which may no longer be absolutely necessary. Once this relationship between the client's conscious self and their inner abandoned child has been turned around, therapeutic work will usually proceed much more smoothly.

CHAPTER 6

Specific Psychotherapeutic Interventions

I will now address the question of specific approaches that I have found especially valuable in the therapy of adults who have been ignored children. The list does not claim to be anything like complete; for myself, I hope to learn many more interventions that help my ignored children clients. Generally speaking, there is a dearth of therapeutic approaches that have been specifically tailored to clients with developmental deficits, and I think it must be a growth area. In the following I will share what I have learned to date.

• My own training background is in body psychotherapy (Hartley, 2009; Staunton, 2002), and this can be adapted to work with clients who have been ignored children. I will describe at some length those elements of body psychotherapy that I have found helpful. As I have outlined in Chapter 3, body psychotherapy is well placed to address the sense of being overstretched that characterizes so many ignored children. Having said this, I want to emphasize that it is not necessary to work directly with the body with ignored children, and often it is not indicated. I have observed many skilled therapists using all sorts of approaches over the years, and usually found that they do similar things as I do, just in different ways. For many clients who were ignored children, working with the body is a way of accessing a deeper level of internal experience that obviates the burden of having to find words. Ignored children are often at their best floating in an undefined and unstructured space where the demands of verbally making themselves understood are not pressing.

- I will discuss finding words and using language to describe experiences, which I think is a tremendously important approach for clients who often struggle to do this.

- I will make a case for finding a narrative of the client's history, especially a narrative that accounts for their current struggles, as a part of therapy—a narrative that can lighten the shame and sense of being lost for ignored children.

- A further section will explore trauma therapy approaches and how they can be used with ignored children to prepare the ground for the developmental deficits to fill in.

- An important part of the therapy for ignored children is support for good feelings. Expressions of praise, appreciation, and love from parental figures have often been nonexistent in their early lives and may actually feel dangerous or otherwise difficult to cope with. If ignored children are to grow into healthy people with healthy self-confidence, this will need addressing.

- Finally, I will make a case for using approaches that stimulate the imagination as perhaps some of the best approaches that the therapeutic world has come up with for the nourishing of the soul, so necessary to ignored children.

In a typical course of therapy with a client who has been an ignored child, I often start by addressing the anxiety and stress that so disables ignored children. In order for the therapeutic process to become easier, it is often a useful first stage to help the client regulate their feelings better. This generally can be expected to create a good experience for the client relatively quickly, and the sense that the therapy is working supports the client's motivation for carrying on. Some body psycho-therapeutic approaches are helpful in this respect, as well as general anxiety and stress-management approaches.

Once anxiety levels and general self-regulation are a little improved, I may in a second stage use a trauma approach to directly address both early (attachment) and incidental trauma. I find that once the baseline of anxiety that results from trauma has been lowered, for example by EMDR, many deficits that were previously impossible to overcome will spontaneously start to fill up. Clients may gradually experience more inner calm, better interpersonal relationships, more self-compassion, a clearer sense of who they are and what they want to do with their lives, and better access to their creativity.

In a third stage I may like to use an approach that starts with an aspect of nonverbal experience. Ignored children often like these, because they play to their strengths and meet them where they are. So I may then choose to do bodywork, or massage, or work with images, or with the creative arts. I think it quite important when using such approaches to keep creating links with language and conscious thought, so that a degree of integration between thoughts and feelings is part of the process and will automatically anchor new material in more than one level of experience.

This will create a lengthy stage of therapy during which whatever material the client brings can be deepened and explored. I will aim to make this pleasurable and supportive, so that it can also serve as a lengthy recovery phase for the client during which they can experience more holding and support than they are likely to have experienced as children and can learn to access some good feelings. Throughout, I will keep in mind that the work of *deficit filling* during this stage will take time. During this process, many dilemmas and conflicts can get explored, and difficulties of present-day life can be addressed.

While it is not my main focus during this stage of therapy, I am aware that gradually this stage needs to flow into a stage in which specific maladaptive coping strategies can be addressed more directly, if the client and I both feel that they are getting in the way. During this fourth stage, I may also go back to trauma approaches if I judge it appropriate. Usually, stages three and four interweave with each other, depending on where I feel that it is possible to progress.

Finally, there will be a fifth stage of therapy, in which the emphasis is on reviewing the process. In this stage, I feel that the most important point is making sure that the client gets to keep all the new resources that we have put in place, as we prepare for ending the therapy.

This type of sequence is a typical treatment plan but not in any way set in stone. Some clients come to therapy specifically asking for body-work, imagery work, or trauma work, and I will usually try to go with this, at least until we hit serious obstacles. The plan outlined above is the kind of sequence that I may follow when presented with a client who was an ignored child and looks to me to provide a plan for them to get better.

Body Psychotherapeutic Approaches

Most gentle body psychotherapeutic techniques can be used to access early material. These include biodynamic massage and vegetotherapy, a technique that is used with variations by most biodynamic, biosynthesis and neo-Reichian psychotherapists (Boadella, 1987; Cimini & Ferri, 2010; Reich, 1972; Southwell, 1988). I apologize to all my body psychotherapist colleagues for my inability to adequately render their wonderful and very subtle work, but for the purpose of this discussion I will focus on the elements all these variations of vegetotherapy have in common. They usually involve the client lying down and being encouraged to be aware of their body sensations, including body sensations that may be evoked by a light touch. Gradually body sensations evolve into feelings, thoughts, and movements. The sessions conducted within this framework ideally evolve into a dialogue that includes a strong element of nonverbal communication—sometimes such sessions can be entirely wordless, although most practitioners will invite the client to reflect on what has happened and to create a meaning out of the experience. Because the client is lying down, and because the focus is on body sensation rather than thought, we can easily understand that early material is preferentially accessed in this context. Often it will be preverbal material, or material that while not originating from preverbal times has not been put into words before.

Biodynamic massage can be used in a very similar way. It is a usually gentle massage aimed at improving self-regulation in the client and almost invariably results over a period of time in better body awareness of the client. Many clients who were ignored children prefer massage to vegetotherapy, because it frees them of the fear that nothing will happen, with its accompanying shame and sense of responsibility—in massage, the therapist is in charge, and the client does not have to do anything. The degree to which I want to meet this wish or not may determine my choice of whether to offer them massage or vegetotherapy, as a matter of fine-tuning the level of challenge that the client is able to rise to at any given time. Some clients do better if allowed to be very passive and follow my lead, because it frees them from an intolerable burden of making decisions. Others feel belittled by or afraid of the passive position as recipient of a massage or may just prefer to feel a little more in charge of the session.

Especially when the touch used is warm, gentle, and finely attuned to the responses of the client's body, both of these techniques create a contact that feels nurturing and loving to many people and can serve to recapture lost or only-just-glimpsed feelings of safety and bliss in early infancy (Eiden, 1998). Clients who were ignored children will respond to this on a spectrum from enormous bliss and enjoyment to absolute terror or traumatic flashback, so there is no general rule about the therapeutic benefit of these interventions. It is very important for those who habitually use them to do their utmost to ascertain whether the client is really enjoying the touch or only pretending to in order to make the therapist happy; if the client is not enjoying the session, many of these interventions will not be of much benefit or may be countertherapeutic. In order to circumvent this problem, biodynamic massage employs a nonverbal feedback tool, the borborygmi (stomach rumbles) of the client, as an additional gauge for how comfortable the touch is at a more unconscious level (Carroll, 2002). Other approaches use breathing and the close observation of the client's body in similar ways.

These body psychotherapeutic approaches can be said to slip underneath the client's resistance and underneath much of their ego defenses—and this is both the great advantage and the great danger of these approaches. The advantage is that clients who were ignored children and who normally offer fierce resistance to therapeutic change may not have the same response to these gentle and pleasant bodily interventions. It may thus be possible for a skilled therapist to gain access to the deeper layer of the ignored child where the—usually very young—child is just lost, terrified, and yearning to be held and made safe. The great danger is that such an experience may be tangled up with traumatic memories that cannot be processed. In that case, the traumatic material may well overwhelm the client and make it impossible for them to benefit from this approach and from the hoped-for healing experience of being cherished and looked after. Instead, such experiences may further fragment the client's experience of themselves by creating more split self-states that cannot be integrated. Realistically it is not possible to predict with any accuracy whether this will happen in any given case, and therefore the therapist may just have to take the risk.

To mitigate the danger, most therapists include an element of translating the experience of being touched into words and attempting to integrate it with conscious thought and the present-day identity of the client. If all of this goes well, then these approaches can be a tremendous benefit in building integration among sensation, feeling, and thought and thus help clients live richer and far more resourced lives than hitherto. Whole seams of inner aliveness and creativity may be accessed, and clients can recover from lifelong depression.

If this type of therapy does not go well, clients may feel that the therapy "didn't do anything for them" and move on without further thought. Or they may feel that the therapy has damaged them by opening up chasms in their personality structure that were well-managed before, thus leaving them open to external and internal attacks, insatiable longings, and unmanageable suffering. Sadly, there is a real risk of this state of mind resulting from body psychotherapy. It has deterred both clients and body psychotherapists from making use of the potential of body psychotherapeutic approaches.

Most often, these body psychotherapeutic approaches are experienced as pleasant by clients, and a philosophy of a "corrective experience" has been built around them by some practitioners. Providing a corrective experience is understood as creating a glimpse of a better experience of life than the client has had hitherto. In this way, the therapist offers the client a chance to change for the better (Castonguay & Hill, 2012). On the other hand, some practitioners of different therapeutic modalities feel strongly that these approaches are essentially a gratification of the client's needs and as such not the job of a psycho-therapist. Moreover, there is a fear that if psychotherapists attempt to provide such corrective experiences, malignant regression is invited; the reasoning is that the client will have no motivation to develop fur-ther if their early needs are being gratified. The belief underlying this fear is that growth happens as a result of challenge and frustration, and therefore by avoiding these we spoil our clients and prevent them from developing a stronger ego.

I take this argument seriously and think that the question may need to be decided on a case-by-case basis. The therapist's experience of their own therapy as well as their general beliefs will influence their decision. In addition, the client's expectations of therapy and the rela-tional pairing between therapist and client needs to be taken into con-sideration. The following are my more general considerations:

I consider it as by no means given that gratification of the client's needs, or just creating an experience that is different from what they are used to, is therapeutic in itself. However, it seems to me that experi-ences of having what we need can under favorable circumstances serve as a foundation on which to rebuild our personality.

With regard to what is often seen as the alternative—namely to frus-trate clients' needs—it seems to me that frustration is a challenge, and every challenge needs to be evaluated in terms of whether the client can make use of it. If they can't, it was too much and needs to be dosed down. Typically, clients who have been ignored children have experi-enced too much challenge and too much frustration, to an extent that they were overwhelmed, or close to overwhelmed. Being overwhelmed, they have not been able to grow, because their brains have been flooded with stress-related hormones that stunt growth. They therefore need to be treated with gentleness until their brains and bodies have recovered from this constant overwhelm.

In addition, the nature of the client's response to a challenge needs to be observed closely: if a challenge leads to the establishment of traumatic defenses or to a state of greater fragmentation, then challenging is contraindicated. On the other hand, if a client is able to make use of challenges, and especially if the therapist is skilled enough to present these in small enough doses that they are still surmountable, they will likely create an experience of success and therefore stimulate growth.

In addition, I would argue that a degree of gratification is a possible intervention if a client has a high resistance against getting better in therapy, as many ignored children do. The philosophy of this approach would be to use the gratification as an experiment. Gratifying some of the client's needs will enable us to observe how the resulting good feelings are warded off. Then the mechanism that gets in the way of therapeutic improvement can be unpacked and explored in the therapy. In this way, we have a real chance of changing how clients receive therapy and make it part of themselves. The mere feeding back to ignored children that they are resisting therapy, or the search for secondary gain motivations, is unlikely to be a successful strategy for this issue; in my experience it needs to be addressed and will not go away by itself.

Finally, much of psychotherapy relies on the observation of client's responses and the reflection on these. To that end, whether a need of the client's is being gratified or frustrated does not in itself matter a very great deal, except if either possibility tends to lead to a habitual loss of the client's ability to reflect, which would then need to be explored further.

Both biodynamic massage and vegetotherapy are specialized psychotherapy techniques that are taught as part of full-length body psychotherapy trainings. In some places, biodynamic massage is also taught as a stand-alone, complementary therapy. Experience with this type of training suggests that biodynamic massage integrates quite well with many psychotherapy approaches, for example Jungian, gestalt, integrative, humanistic, or attachment-based psychotherapies. For psychotherapists not trained in the use of these techniques, referring the client to a colleague who is may be an option. Alternatively, asking the client to see a biodynamic massage therapist concomitantly with non-body-based psychotherapy may also be an option. Working in other ways that create greater well-being and safety for the client to be in their own body is also possible.

The other major body psychotherapy modality to be mentioned here is relational trauma therapy, an approach arising mostly out of the Bodynamic Analysis school in Copenhagen. Relational trauma therapy is the work of Merete Holm Brantbjerg who currently teaches in Denmark, Sweden, the UK, and the Netherlands. Relational trauma therapy has been developed with a specific focus on the role of hypo-responsive muscles and hypo-arousal as part of trauma patterns, but it applies equally to developmental deficits in general.

Hypo-responsive muscles are usually the result of a developmental arrest in the early stage of the developmental phase during which normally the function of a particular muscle or muscle group is acquired. In this early stage of a developmental phase, a new movement has just become possible through the acquisition of voluntary control over the relevant muscles. Because it is new, the movement is going to be quite tentative at first. This contrasts with the same movement in the late stage of the developmental phase, when the child has become really enthusiastic about the new capability and is practicing the movement over and over again. In the early stage, a child can easily be discouraged from engaging with a new movement and will then refrain from doing so. The result of such an event is the emergence of a deficit relating to this movement. In the body of an adult, this may well manifest as a lack of tone, or a low-energy state, of the relevant muscle group.

Hypo-responsive muscles are thus the physical correlate of developmental deficits in psychological functioning and, like their psychological counterparts, represent a paucity of resources for the regulation and containment of the person's emotional and physical life. This leaves the person more at the mercy of the outside world than others with more muscle tone and more psychological resources. In normal development, we can assume that there will be a number of movements that are well developed and others that are underdeveloped. Therefore every person will be a mixture of hyper- and hypo-responsive muscles, as well as balanced, filled-out muscles; to an extent, every individual will have their own individual pattern of anatomical distribution between hyper- and hypo-responsive muscles. Extreme conditions in a child's early life can lead to an extreme preponderance of either hyper-responsive or hypo-responsive muscles. In some traumatized states, extremes of either hyper-responsive muscles (in a state called tonic immobility) or hypo-responsive muscles (collapse into passivity) can become very generalized (see Rothschild, 2017).

I am mostly interested here in the aspect of relational trauma therapy that addresses hypo-responsive muscles and muscle groups resulting from developmental deficit. By feeling our own bodies or observing those of others, we can become aware of the movements that involve hypo-responsive muscles, although this is usually more difficult than becoming aware of tension and hyper-responsive muscles. Activating hypo-responsive muscles may feel like hard work, or feel unfamiliar and strange, or feel downright uncomfortable or scary. We may have a strong sense that we "don't want to go there."

When we explore hypo-responsive muscle with clients, it can happen that they encounter a muscle or a movement that is part of a somatic marker for a traumatic memory. In that case the client can feel nauseated or spaced out. It is nearly always a good idea to balance using a hypo-responsive muscle with using a well-developed one—often the opposite movement is mediated by well-toned or hyper-responsive muscles. So, for example, if a client feels uncomfortable pushing something or somebody away from themselves by extending their elbows (using their elbow extensor muscles, chiefly triceps), there are two possibilities for modifying the exercise. We can try to encourage them to experiment with pushing less strongly and in that way dose down the movement. If they can find a degree of pushing that feels comfortable and good, there will be a spontaneous rebalancing of the muscles. If they cannot reach this point, then it may be better to ask them to pull toward themselves by flexing their elbows (using their elbow flexor muscles, chiefly biceps), until the uncomfortable feeling has abated.

Relational trauma therapy integrates an awareness of power dynamics into the bodily interventions and is thus particularly suitable for ignored children who typically feel terribly shamed by their perceived inadequacies and by needing therapy. The approach meets and contains these feelings in a solid therapeutic relationship, noting as a matter of fact when an intervention is unsuitable for a particular body structure without attaching a value judgment to that. As the whole therapeutic approach is resource-oriented, it is very well suited for clients with developmental deficits that need filling in. In the relational context created, muscles can be explored to determine which ones are available and responsive and which ones do not respond so well and need smaller challenges. Finding the right dose of challenge for any particular muscle can then be felt as a profoundly satisfying experience that will lead on to more confidence and an expansion of the whole personality. Once such a right dose of challenge has been found, the competitiveness and one-upmanship often associated with striving for high-energy states becomes much less important and the person can develop at their own pace and in their own way much more easily.

Relational trauma therapy is more movement-based and places less emphasis on touch and on the therapist as a reparenting figure than other body psychotherapy approaches. The work requires tremendous skill in holding the space in which this very detailed and slow exploration can take place fruitfully. It also requires a good knowledge of psychomotor development. I would not advise therapists to attempt to do it without any training. However, there is a manual of presence skills that is publicly available. Presence skills are bodily skills that support a therapist's presence; most of them are also suitable for use with clients and can become valuable resources (Moaiku, 2019). Relational trauma therapy offers different ways of doing every movement or exercise and thus makes it possible for each client to find the one that works best for them individually.

Pearl often complains that when somebody wants something from her, she loses her sense of self and goes on autopilot, usually responding with "yes." After spending a lot of time unravelling the history of this reflex response, and understanding how it has served her in the past and still does, we both agree that she has reached a new state of self-possession and could start to experiment with different responses. It is at this point that we want to address the mechanics of this type of situation, in order to give her a chance of catching what exactly is happening and seeing what her options might be. I try to help her develop some ways of supporting her self-possession by physically strengthening the connection with her core and hopefully setting cues for a pause for thought.

I therefore select an exercise, one of a series that Holm Brantbjerg calls presence skills. The first one is to simply sit and feel her feet on the floor and her back against the chair. Then I suggest pushing her feet a little bit into the floor. She pushes willingly, but then makes a face and says, "Oh dear, that just shows up how unfit I am—I think this will be too tiring for me." I suggest she push less and keep reducing the push until she can't feel herself pushing any more. Then I say, "Now just give the smallest push that you can." Her face clears, and she takes a deeper breath, saying, "Ah, yes, that's much better. Now it feels comfortable." I make sure she can let the tension from the push travel up her body and feel it supporting her.

I encourage her to experiment with putting her weight more on the inside of her feet and outside of her feet. I ask if she can feel a difference and get her to describe the different sensations in words. With her weight on the medial half of her feet, she feels her belly more and experiences this as very calming and centering. With her weight on the lateral half of her feet, she is more aware of her back and the strength in it. As she says this, she increases the pressure on her feet a little and starts to smile. "This is lovely—I feel really strong now. I could say no to anybody in this position!"

Relational trauma therapy supports my experience that there is no one-size-fits-all in using the physical body to help create resources for clients in low-energy states. Rather, finding body-based resources that are helpful for clients needs to be a joint exploration, with the therapist able to provide a range of possibilities. I am extremely grateful to Babette Rothschild for formulating that many people who suffer from PTSD experience difficulties when they try to use run-of-the-mill mindfulness approaches or attempt to calm themselves down by breathing or body awareness (Rothschild, 2017). It is important for therapists who want to work in such ways to have a large repertoire of possible interventions, as well as a creative mind that can invent new ones if necessary.

Words and Language

Words are powerful containers. Arguably they are an important healing ingredient of most if not all psychotherapies. A person who lacks the ability to put their inner world into words is extremely vulnerable to the vagaries of other people's ability to tune into their nonverbal communication and to being used as a canvas for others on which to project their own inner dynamic. It will thus be difficult for such a person to develop a sense of identity separate from other people. They will also find that their range of possible communications with others is extremely limited. Moreover, their experience of their own inner world may be severely curtailed and impoverished. For such a person, to acquire the ability to put feelings into words presents an immeasurable benefit that will transform their life.

While it has been argued that 93% of human communication is nonverbal (Mehrabian & Ferris, 1967), nevertheless verbal communication is crucial (Lapakko, 1997). Only words can mitigate at least partly against misunderstandings that may prove fatal to human relationships. Language is an important ego function. Thoughts can usually be put into words, even if sometimes not with a high degree of fidelity. It is very hard to imagine a person having some kind of reflective ability without words and language. The development of a healthy acting and containing ego depends crucially on the development of an ability to symbolize experience in language.

Clients who have been ignored children often struggle to find words for their internal experience. This may have multiple reasons such as high anxiety, crippling shame, or the fear of exposing themselves, as well as various relational difficulties; there may also be deficits arising directly from the neglect they have suffered. In addition, many ignored children have a poor ability to put feelings and words together. Those who have not learned to name different feelings or have not learned what the bodily experience of these feelings is may be labelled alexithymic. In some cases there may be genetic mutations, epigenetic changes, or perhaps brain injuries to account for this. However, mostly we can see it as a sign of the neglect these clients have suffered: nobody has taken the trouble to help them experience different feelings and then put words to them, so that the feelings become familiar, describable, and containable. For such clients, feelings are almost inevitably overwhelming. I have heard statements from clients such as, *It just feels like a black wave that engulfs me*, or, *I can't find any words for this—I know there are feelings there but I can't tell what they are.*

In therapy such clients may be told that they are split off from their feelings and need to connect more with their emotions. Unfortunately, attempts to connect thought and feeling more will almost inevitably re-traumatize these clients, as the reason they disconnected their thoughts from their feelings in the first place is that the feelings were overwhelming. If these clients are lucky, they will be confident enough (or stubborn enough) to make their therapists understand that they are out of touch with their emotions for a good reason.

The inability to put words and feelings together can be seen as a big developmental deficit that is typical for ignored children and may need filling in as part of the therapy. As therapists, we have to help our clients put body sensations, emotions, and words together in such a way that the result creates an internally felt connection for the client. This will inevitably be a good experience if we get it right, like something clicking into place typically generating a sense of relief or even pleasure.

It is important for this type of work to happen in a spirit of experimentation. In this way it avoids becoming a demand to the client and allows them to really focus on their own felt sense. I have found that if I am reasonably well-attuned to a client, I can often make a guess as to what they might be feeling and then ask them to see whether that fits. Quite often I will make several suggestions, because many clients find it much easier to pick the best fit out of a range of words describing feelings rather than deciding whether a word I suggest is a good fit or not. Offering several suggestions also helps untangle any relational complications out of this therapeutic exchange, since it is difficult for the client to think they get it wrong. It will thus help keep the anxiety levels low and preserve the client's best ability to think and learn. Most importantly, offering several suggestions allows for the client to start with an approximation to their feeling that can later on be improved as either of us thinks of a better word.

Another help may be to have an image of a feeling. A client might start with one image and in time develop modifications, or different images, as their ability to feel and contain different emotions grows. Asking whether a feeling is a good feeling or a bad one is also helpful—any way to describe feelings is helpful. A location in the body may be good if the client can feel their body in some way. Or there may be a sound without words, or a gesture or movement, that characterizes a feeling.

In order to do this type of work, it is necessary for there to be an understanding between the therapist and the client that this is a difficulty, and there should be some motivation on the part of the client to develop a better range of emotional articulation. Working at such a level of detail cannot otherwise be easily understood by clients. The benefits of attending to this task whenever an opportunity offers are tremendous and will include better resilience to stress, not so much diffuse anxiety, and often a better appreciation of books, poetry, and other art forms that rely on a person's ability to resonate emotionally with words.

Mortimer is an example of this type of neglect. If I ask him how he feels, he typically can't tell me. I take that seriously, and it seems to me to be the result of a combination of factors: he has clearly learned to edit out anxious feelings and not be aware of them; and my questions after how he feels put him on the spot, so that he freezes and loses the ability to put his experience into words. Apart from these factors, it is also clear that his parents took it for granted that he would know what feelings were and would be able to name them. It just didn't occur to them that a small child might need to learn this.

Mortimer has been told that he needs to have more feelings—particularly his girlfriend tells him this. He is therefore motivated to become more emotionally literate. Sometimes I see a change in him that suggests an emotion: his eyes might well up a little, or a faint blush might spread over his face, or the tissues in his face might become a little puffy. I work initially to just note when this happens, so that we can both agree that there is a feeling there. Then I give him a list of possibilities. We are both very pleased when it turns out that he can pick the best fit out of such a list.

A further conversation elicits that he does recognize two emotions in himself: anxiety and shame. He tells me one day that this already a sign of tremendous progress: it took him until he was nearly 20 years old to realize that he had been anxious all his life. He thinks that his parents deliberately didn't tell him he was anxious because they thought he would feel this was a problem and get even more anxious. While we can both understand their reasons and appreciate the good intentions behind them, we also note that this left him floundering on his own for longer than he might have had to. He surprises me at this point in our conversation by saying, "Sometimes I feel so full of anger that I want to shout at them. I was struggling and they made it worse, and that's not okay." This is the first time he names a feeling without being prompted. What's more, the feeling creates a move to separate from his parents and marks the beginning of a separation that Mortimer needs to go through in order to become his own person.

This example also illustrates that the integration of words with feelings and body sensations is an important step in the creation of a narrative of the client's inner world, of their story, that makes it possible for them to connect with other people by letting them know what it is like inside themselves. Not only does this produce a very powerful container for a person's sense of who they are, but it also facilitates supportive and empathic contact with others. It can be the beginning of a move away from the compulsive caregiver personality so common among clients who were ignored children.

Creating Narrative

One of the big obstacles for adults who were ignored children to access therapy is their lack of a narrative of how they came to be as they are. It is perhaps the commonest presentation that they will say there is no history of anything wrong. Their childhood was fine, nothing really bad has ever happened. They simply don't understand why they are suffering as much as they are, and they think they must just be stupid. Some come up with particularly punitive suggestions such as, "I was spoiled and need challenging," or "I am lazy," or "I let myself down all the time in order for people to feel sorry for me." Such self-accusations are widespread among clients who were ignored children, little bits of testimony to the power of the introjected early experiences or possibly the legacies of unsuccessful attempts at therapy.

This presentation results likely from a combination of the fact that neglect is generally hidden and lacks recognition as a serious cause of human suffering and of the difficulty that ignored children have in putting their subjective experience into words. Having never been encouraged to do so, they mostly grow up lonely and without other people who want to know what their experience is and share their own. It is difficult to overstate the devastation that this isolation causes in the mind of a young human being.

While we can make efforts to have emotional neglect more publicly recognized as a serious problem, we also need to help our ignored children clients find their own narrative to account for their difficulties to their own satisfaction. I have often seen how transformative it is for them to feel that not only can they be understood by others, but they can also understand themselves. It diminishes shame and the identification with the perpetrators—the neglectful caregivers. It gives people hope that things may change and the self-confidence to try to make change happen. Many clients find that it paves the way for a more empathic relationship with their own inner child. Following on from the previous section of this chapter, it provides a very powerful container for nebulous and poorly containable feelings.

Some of the creation of narrative can consist of psychoeducation. We can tell our clients about what is known, particularly in the attachment world, about the lack of early attunement. The number of self-help books available on the topic is growing rapidly. Other materials are more dramatic: for example, I have sometimes played footage from Ed Tronick's Still Face experiments to clients (Tronick, 2009). My experience is that such footage is a powerful way to illustrate what clients may struggle to understand, but it can be disturbing if clients connect to the children who get abandoned in this way. I therefore take care to show this footage to clients in a session rather than ask them to watch it at home. Other pieces of psychoeducation that may be useful could be the function of the autonomic nervous system (ANS), which often helps people to manage anxiety more effectively; the existence of the social engagement system and how to activate it; or basic attachment theory.

From an attachment perspective, the co-creation of a narrative for the client's difficulties also forms part of a process of attachment. The point at which the client can take ownership of their own story may well be a sign that they are growing their own identity and becoming more powerful in their own right, rather than continuing to be dependent on the expertise of the therapist as a container and caregiver. It will facilitate the separation from the therapist necessary for completing therapy if the client can take their own narrative with them and elaborate it further on their own.

Often with clients who were ignored children, it is difficult to create a narrative of what has gone wrong in their lives because they are so insecurely attached and need to protect their early caregivers so strongly. This means that they will resist any narrative that even appears to lay any part of the responsibility for their symptoms on their caregivers. In effect, they will live with the narrative of their caregivers about their lives, rather than their own. This creates massive problems: not only does it perpetuate an already enmeshed relationship, but it also makes it hard for an ignored child to have a clear identity.

Working toward the creation of a narrative that accounts for the present-day difficulties that these clients are experiencing may thus need to be embedded in the general work of helping them become a more separate and independent being. This difficulty illustrates how the therapeutic process of ignored children can resemble the inching forward of several strands of a weave, where progress can only ever be made a tiny amount at a time on each strand, and then all the other strands need to be readjusted, because they all interact with each other very tightly and progress on each of them is dependent on progress on all the others.

Most people who have had some therapy know that each time they recount difficult experiences in contact with others, the emotional pain lessens a little. In addition, I would argue that the creation of a narrative that encompasses the client's life history is deeply soul-building (White, 2007). Having a narrative about who we are provides us with a hugely important resource that allows a felt sense of self and an identity to be built on. This makes it an important step in the filling in of developmental deficits.

Of all my clients, Pearl has shown the least interest in her history and always wanted to focus on the future, on getting better. I have followed her in this without asking too many questions. We skirt around the edges of her history, shedding light on little bits of it here and there. After many sessions of this, Pearl is already much better able to tolerate not caregiving all the time, and we are working toward the end of her therapy. One day I allude accidentally to the story she has told me very early on, that her mother rejected her for being a girl when she was born. I say something like "No wonder you need to earn your place in the world constantly by caring for others, seeing how your mother rejected you at birth." It is as if a lightbulb has switched itself on in her head at that moment. She is putting these two things together for the first time ever and staggers at the realization that they form, indeed, a central pillar of the narrative of her life. In a flash, she sees how underneath the need to care for everybody and not abandon anybody, there is the unbearable pain of a baby who has been rejected by her mother in the first moments of her life. She can actually taste the utter panic in the face of this void that must have engulfed her baby self.

Luckily this happens in the middle of a session, so we have some time to sit with her new realization. I help her to make a space for it in her body, and keep reminding her that she survived this and is alive now.

The following week she comes in looking radiant. "Now I can end therapy," she says, "because now I understand why I am as I am. I am a proper person now with a reason to be as she is, and I can tell other people that reason. I feel much more in charge of my life, and I think I will be able to make changes more easily now."

Some clients who were ignored children have very fragmented autobiographical memories, particularly from their early lives, or memories with large gaps in them. Most therapists would think of these clients as the more traumatized of ignored children. Creating a coherent autobiographical timeline of their lives is usually felt as greatly healing for these clients. It may reduce their inner chaos, and they may gain a level of control over their impulses and actions that they may not have known previously. I have had several clients who have drawn or painted internal maps of how they have developed on paper, "just to show you." Some of these were awe-inspiring works of art, and all were infinitely useful in the further course of therapy. Apart from such creative moments, I have generally observed that any work with the autobiographical narrative of ignored children is felt as nurturing and supportive and constitutes a very gentle way of being seen that does not leave clients feeling exposed or invaded but feeling valued and taken seriously.

Finally, I have worked with clients who were ignored children who, as we went along, developed a narrative of how the therapy worked and what it was doing. My impression is that this was a good thing for these clients: they clearly enjoyed the sense of agency and empowerment that came through doing it. It helped build self-confidence as they were able to shift from seeing therapy as a shameful punishment to seeing it as an achievement to be proud of. It was also clearly an achievement in finding words for processes that started out a bit mysterious and gradually became more clearly discernible, like a landscape rising out of mist.

Over time, this process has contributed to establishing an internal therapist for these clients, an internalized good object that they could rely on to remind them of their resources if they became overwhelmed in daily life. The internal therapist kept on existing in their minds long after the end of therapy.

Trauma Approaches

I have made the point elsewhere that neglected people are traumatized and recognizable as such, although the symptoms are subtly different, resembling more the symptoms of burnout than the symptoms of more classical PTSD. Following this thought, it seems possible to work with trauma-based approaches to address the neglect. My tendency to follow such a course has grown, at least in part, out of curiosity to see whether reducing the traumatization in the nervous system would result in a degree of spontaneous filling in of developmental deficits. This follows my theory that the human psyche is extremely resilient and will tend to get what it needs from wherever it is available. If it doesn't, it's a safe assumption that there must be something preventing it. Trauma is a likely candidate for such a block to a spontaneous healing process.

The rationale for using trauma approaches is also that some deficits do have conflicts at their root, just as some conflicts have deficits at their roots. I find that for some clients it really isn't possible to find conflicts that, when resolved, will alleviate anxiety substantially; but this is not always the case. Trauma approaches, including the so-called early trauma approaches, can make it possible to see the conflicts that were previously shrouded in the nebulosity of generalized anxiety.

Many trauma approaches use body sensations as an important element. For some ignored children this may be a stumbling block as they may be reluctant to get in touch with their body sensations, reluctant to move, and reluctant to experiment with doing therapy in any way other than sitting in a chair. Having said that, there are body-based interventions that are usually well tolerated and can be used with even reluctant clients as experiments. It may be worthwhile to start with some body-based interventions that are aimed at providing stability and more resources for clients, because these often reduce the barriers to body awareness greatly, besides being rather fun to do. Such interventions typically involve contacting strength and confidence in the body by gently tensing particularly strong muscles or making movements that cue particularly resourced ego states or particularly powerful images (Rothschild, 2004). One of my favorite exercises, which I learned from David Boadella, is getting clients to push slightly outwards with their arms as they inhale (what is termed an "inbreath") while visualizing breathing in more space for themselves to be who they are. Once clients have contacted these good and supportive body sensations, they will often feel much braver about using body sensation in other ways later on. It is a good rule of thumb to do any movements on an inbreath (or as "counterpulsation"), because this feels containing and does not generally encourage any type of catharsis that might overwhelm the client.

For clients who cannot feel their bodies, it is sometimes possible to pretend that they do and make up body sensations. This can be elicited by the therapist by asking things like, "If you were to feel this somewhere in your body, where do you think it might be?" or simply by asking them to guess at body sensations. Such guesses are likely to be not far off, and the maneuver will take some pressure off the client.

In terms of actual processing of traumatic memories, appropriate memories to choose for clients who have been ignored children may include adverse events that they can remember. Examples of these might be being bullied (which is common among ignored children) or being otherwise maltreated because they couldn't set up adequate boundaries or protect themselves. Some clients have memories of instances when the neglect was clearly experienced including the associated distress of feeling abandoned and helpless. There may also be memories of being misunderstood, blamed, or humiliated. All these can be worked through and will decrease the client's background anxiety and vulnerability to stress.

For my own practice, it has been transformative to learn EMDR (Shapiro, 2001) and particularly to learn the EMDR early trauma approaches. I have found that these approaches (see for example O'Shea, 2009; Paulsen, 2017) make the therapy of adults who were ignored children much quicker by reducing a baseline level of anxiety that otherwise acts rather like a strong headwind on a cyclist, rendering the work more time- and energy-consuming.

In early trauma EMDR, we attempt to process memories that are present only implicitly in the form of somatic markers and have no narrative. We therefore tend to work with imagined targets rather than actual narrative memories. EMDR practitioners that I consult with generally feel that imaginary targets are fine to process if there are no clear, explicit memories. Most of my clients who were ignored children can visualize well and find it quite easy to imagine what their experience in utero or as an infant might have been like. Sometimes they ask whether what they visualize in this way is likely to be what really happened. I generally say that we cannot make any judgments about the relationship between such images and historical fact, but that therapy is uniquely interested in their memories of whatever kind of their early life, as this gives us access to the problems that influence their current life. Therefore from a therapeutic point of view, we can say that what they visualize reflects a subjective truth that is relevant to the therapeutic process. They may need to live with not knowing if what they visualize in this manner actually happened or not.

In my experience there are slight differences between processing imagined targets and processing real memories. The work tends to be rather slower with imagined targets, as such images are more fluid and less clearly defined in the client's mind. It seems important to make sure that what the client visualizes comes with feelings, if possible feelings that can be located in the body. Otherwise the therapy effort is like trying to process something that is quite split off from the person's psyche and may not process at all.

The other main feature of EMDR with early trauma is that we often move the client deliberately to a happier, calmer, and more resourced feeling state by asking them to imagine how they would have needed things to be. This is done when the client appears to get stuck in distressing memories. Again, when asked, I will explain that I am not aiming to change or deny the past but merely attempting to rebalance the client's feelings between distressing and soothing ones and to help them focus on things in their childhood that were good and nurturing and supportive of their development.

I have found it often helpful to combine trauma work with what is called Ego State therapy (Forgash & Copley, 2008), an approach that utilizes a co-constructed model of the client's mind that allows for different self-states (or ego states). I typically get my clients to distinguish among the classical three self-states of Transactional Analysis (parent, adult, and child). However, the construction of these models of mind needs to be highly individualized. Some clients like using more self-states and can distinguish between states of themselves that correspond to different ages and different levels of resources and traumatic experiences. To be able to assign any trauma or traumatic network being worked on to a particular self-state helps to keep it contained. It also makes it easier to finish sessions with the client in a current state and sufficiently resourced to leave my consulting room and negotiate streets and traffic safely. This kind of model also helps clients understand feelings that appear to be wildly inappropriate for current situations but can be located to a particular time in the client's past. These feelings can then be called "emotional flashbacks" (Grannon, 2016) and treated with an appropriate technique, often involving the creation and strengthening of dual awareness. The skills gained in this way allow clients to pull themselves back into the present in real-life situations outside the therapy room and will underpin their sense of being in charge of their own lives. I have generally found that the joint construction of this type of model of their own minds is tremendously helpful for clients who were ignored children and builds much confidence in their own ability to help themselves.

The processing of a client's life just before birth and in the first weeks and months of their lives usually has good effects on their general well-being. Clients tell me that they feel much calmer; they are more able to deal with previously difficult situations and feel more able to "have a normal life."

I offer a piece of early trauma EMDR to Olivia as we discuss her mother giving her up for adoption. Olivia is enthusiastic, because she feels so strongly that this one event has blighted her whole life. I settle her comfortably in her chair and hand her the tactile stimulation device (the "buzzers") that allows me to remain in my chair and not have to invade her space.

I ask her to close her eyes and to go back in her mind to a time before anything went wrong. She quite readily goes back to before she was born, basking in the warmth of her mother's womb and in the feeling of her mother's presence. She dwells a little on her mother's state of mind and says it feels like "her body loved me and was happy I was there, but her mind is full of fears and thoughts that she shouldn't feel like that." I get her to focus on her mother's love for a bit. Then I ask Olivia to move forward in time, and she goes to the time when she has to leave the safe place of her mother's body. Then the catastrophe hits as Olivia has just emerged from her mother's womb and feels her mother's attempt to hold her, but somebody pulls her away from the warmth and safety. She gets a sense of screaming in panic and distress, screaming, screaming. I do another set of bilateral stimulation but she just remains with the screaming image. So I ask her to think about how she would have needed it to be. She gasps, "I needed to be held—I was much too small to cope with this cold and lonely place, it was horrible." I ask her to imagine this. She imagines being tightly held in her mother's arms. I talk to her, reinforcing the safety and warmth of the place, still keeping the bilateral stimulation going, and gradually she calms down. We end the session soon after.

In the next session, she starts by wanting to discuss whether we are "trying to change history." This is not unexpected, and so I explain that I am changing her physical state and trying to set up the ability in herself to change it and that this is the point of the work, not changing her history. We both know that the past has happened and cannot be changed now. Only her feelings about it can change.

Over the next few sessions, we repeat this sequence several times. Each time it changes a little. From her mother's arms, she gradually imagines being in the arms of "a loving person." The degree of distress experienced decreases markedly as she becomes able to remember throughout that she knows the feeling of being held and loved. Gradually she can maintain the sense of her mother's love that she gained from the pre-birth part of the visualization and keep remembering that at least part of her mother loved her and wanted her.

We are very focused on this piece of work, and so I am slightly surprised as she comes in one day after about 6 weeks and tells me that she is sleeping better than she ever has in her life. "This is really working, and it is making a huge difference, although I would struggle to tell you exactly what the difference is." It becomes clearer some months later when she confides that she has fallen in love—and for a change with a man who seems to return her feelings.

Supporting Good Feelings

I want to address two issues in this section. The first is that many clients who were ignored children find it very difficult to let themselves have good feelings. This can make therapeutic progress very arduous if not impossible for them. I want to share specific interventions that can address this difficulty. The second issue is that many ignored children are somewhat solitary, relying on their own resources as they do, and therefore one of their deficits may be the lack of a robust social engagement system. Again, it seems to me that it is worthwhile working to fill in this deficit, at least to an extent.

Clients who were ignored children often feel threatened by feeling better, by making progress in therapy, and by experiencing joy, pride, or excitement at their progress. Feeling threatened may operate on an unconscious level, or they may be aware of it. Only rarely will they also be aware that this is a serious problem. If given positive feedback, or paid a compliment, they will typically brush it aside or deny deserving it. Chapter 5 has addressed at some length my understanding of the possible issues involved in this. The first task for therapists when presented with this observation is usually to try and unravel it in order to understand what the issue is.

There is a belief by practitioners of most body psychotherapy and other humanistic psychotherapy modalities that to experience good feelings is healing. This may not be true for all clients, but for ignored children it certainly is, given how hard they generally find life and how much time they spend just coping and plodding on. Pleasurable feelings switch on the parasympathetic nervous system, and specifically the ventral vagal complex (VVC), more powerfully than anything else. As a consequence, they tend to expand the physical body, encourage us to breathe more deeply, relax many skeletal muscles, increase blood flow to the skin and extremities, and switch the brain to its most resourced state, promoting mature and spacious thinking. The kind of psychophysiological state that is triggered by pleasurable experiences is of tremendous importance. Not only does it provide us with some protection against stress and anxiety; it also promotes the assimilation and integration of any new learning that we may acquire in therapy (Stauffer, 2005).

Therefore the fact that ignored children often seem uncomfortable having good feelings can really get in the way of their recovery. While having this peculiarity understood and taken seriously by an empathic therapist is usually helpful, sometimes that just isn't enough. We may want to train clients' emotional muscle for good feelings, or we may want to help them be aware every time they brush off or dismantle a good feeling, so that they can make choices. Or we simply may want to create more congruence between their presentation to the outside world and their internal feeling state.

Sometimes clients who were ignored children find that their negative self-talk is so powerful and destructive that it swallows up any positive feelings or thoughts that might want to arise. In those cases I tend to work toward establishing some protection against this. I will suggest to the client that we install a benign and protective parental figure who can exist side by side with the critical and destructive parental figure in the client's mind, who points out how destructive the negative self-talk is and how much the client deserves better. Such protective parental figures can have the voices of actual parental figures from the client's life—perhaps a grandparent, or a teacher who was kind, or similar. Alternatively, they can be imagined as very powerful fairy godparents or champion knights in shining armor or patron saints or similar figures of great power. It may be a good idea to install these figures using bilateral stimulation with clients who are used to EMDR. If the client has reached a point at which they are able to experience the full horror of the internalized destruction and can separate from it far enough to see it as undesirable, then there is a chance that this kind of protective figure can help make the destruction less potent.

I have learned a little exercise from Andrew Leeds (2015) to practice taking in positive feedback. It seems gentle enough to me to have a chance of working, simple enough to be easily done, and a small enough intervention to be achievable by most clients. It contains an element of fostering awareness in the client of how their inability to receive positive feedback comes across to others.

I decide one day to teach Pearl this exercise, as part of what we have come to call "receptiveness practice." I first demonstrate to her two possible responses to getting a compliment. I ask her to say something nice to me, and she says "I like your home-knitted socks." The first time she says it, I dismiss the compliment with, "Knitting is just what I do of an evening to relax," not looking at her as I say it. She is struck with how dismissed she feels. The second time she says the same thing, I am careful to maintain eye contact, take a breath into my upper chest in order to create a space for the compliment, smile, and say, "Thank you, I appreciate that." She smiles back at me, and we share a long good moment of mutual appreciation. Then we reverse roles, and I say to her "I like what a good mother you are." The first time, as instructed, she looks away and says "I'm not really—I fail so often." I ask her how she feels. She says she just catches the little tinge of disappointment at letting the compliment slip away from her. I repeat it, and this time she also makes a space for it in her upper chest and keeps looking at me. She gets quite tearful as she does this and lets herself feel how much she has longed to hear this.

This exercise does two things: it helps the client create a space in their body for a good feeling, and it keeps the good feeling in contact with the therapist. This latter aspect will promote the development of a healthier and more active social engagement system. As I have described in Chapter 4, the social engagement system embodies our ability to make use of contact with other people for our benefit. For many clients who were ignored children, this represents a massive shift, because they have grown up regarding other people as the problem, not as the solution. While I have strong feelings about labeling introversion or shyness as in any way pathological, I have come to appreciate the benefits of being able to make use of contact with other people in emotional self-regulation.

The main caveat with this type of exercise is that unless both client and therapist are very clear about what they are doing, it can easily become yet another "should" for a client who is already hedged in by shoulds; thus it can just add to their burden of rules to observe in order to create a semblance of a normal life or to their shame about perceived inadequacies. It seems to me that we can only use this type of intervention in a well-established therapeutic relationship in which we have earned a large amount of relational safety. In addition, I would want to be reasonably certain before doing the exercise that it has a good chance of succeeding, because it is the kind of exercise that can do much good if it succeeds and much damage if it fails. So it is probably an exercise to be brought into the therapy in the later stages of the therapeutic process.

Other interventions are possible to help clients bring awareness to what they do with good feelings, along the lines of actively slowing an experience down and helping the client to go through it with maximum awareness of all aspects of it. For those a light touch on the part of the therapist is required. If a client finds the topic difficult, it may be all we can do to be seemingly indifferent to any therapeutic progress they make in order to improve its chances of becoming well established without the internal destruction mechanism being triggered.

Many therapists like making suggestions for what clients can do in order to be more resourced, enjoy life more, and manage their anxiety better. As with other interventions, ignored children will need accurate dosing of encouragement to look after themselves better and do more things that will make them feel good. Lifestyle changes are especially difficult and possibly more so for ignored children, who are generally not used to easily changing anything at all in their lives. So for the therapist to negotiate between what would be ideal and what is possible is good practice. Therapists should also be aware of the danger of getting locked in an enactment in which they are trying to make the client do something that the client resists because they feel unable to do it. With ignored children, perhaps more than with other clients, it is important always to keep in mind that when working with issues of client self-care, we are dealing with serious conflicts; therapists should hold both sides of the conflict in mind and not take sides in a way that feels attacking to the client.

Particularly the humanistic psychotherapies, and latterly also the relational psychoanalytical psychotherapies, have always cherished the belief that the therapeutic relationship itself can serve as the vehicle for building a more highly functioning social engagement system. Generally the assumption is that this works even if it is not explicitly named or consciously experienced by the client, as therapist and client will co-regulate to an extent when in proximity to each other. However, I think when working with clients who have been ignored children, we need to take into account that they may experience any contact with others as hard work, frightening, and stressful, and these feelings may undermine the normal relational effect of psychotherapy. Especially if the therapist has an investment in being seen (and seeing themselves) as a good person and a good therapist, ignored children will then simply gratify this wish of the therapist's without necessarily gaining any benefit for themselves. I therefore think that when working with clients who were ignored children, therapists need to be open to the possibility that their presence may not in itself be very therapeutic in the early stages of therapy. They will have to be able to bear this realization without feeling destroyed and retaliating, and they may need to go for a long time without getting much positive feedback from the client.

Having said that, clients who were ignored children are human beings and will therefore draw some benefit from regular contact with a benign therapist. If the therapist is thoroughly attentive to the creation of safety for the individual client, the relationship is likely to work even better. The process of building safety works in a similar way as the process of managing anxiety: the more work you have already done, the easier it becomes and the faster progress is made. The reason is that both types of strategies work best when the arousal in the sympathetic nervous system (SNS) is low, and the lower it gets over time, the more effective interventions to lower it further will become. This underpins, once more, that to find ways of monitoring a client's ANS state is of crucial importance when working with clients who may not be able to self-report accurately.

The kinds of interventions that I might choose to use with ignored children in order to build more good feelings in a relationship are varied. Laughing and having fun together works very well. Some of my best strategies for cueing a client's here-and-now adult self-state involve having fun together—for instance throwing cushions at each other, or playing with a balloon, or jumping up and down together, or pushing the soles of our feet against each other. Therapists will do well to get their creativity going for this purpose! Every client is different, and every therapist has different ideas of what could be done to have fun together, and so every therapist-client pair needs to negotiate the best ways of building the fun part of their relationship. Choosing some kind of physical activity has advantages (although it may not be possible for some clients or therapists) in that it helps to get the clients into their bodies more. Laughing and smiling together at things that both find funny is often easier and also works well when done sensitively. Co-creating a work of art is also a good option.

I will also strongly encourage ignored children to build ways of sharing enjoyment into other relationships in their lives. This is partly because 1 hour a week is not enough to counteract all the effects of a stressful and frightening life and partly because I do not want to foster the belief that I am the only person in my clients' lives who is good for them. On the contrary, I am aiming to create more openness in my clients' minds for the possibility that, frightening though many people may be, there are some out there who are safe and can be enjoyable to be with.

Imaginal Work

In my mind, work with imagery holds a special place in the therapy world as perhaps the most effective soul-building approach. It is not coincidence that psychosynthesis, which explicitly names itself in antithesis to psychoanalysis, wanting to build rather than dismantle, uses imagery very freely (Assagioli, 1999; Ferrucci, 1982). Various submodalities of body psychotherapy also make extensive use of imagery, particularly images arising out of body sensations (Landale, 2002). Images are powerful containers and often act as guiding stars for clients' lives, illuminating a perspective into the future. My own therapeutic journey started with imagery (Leuner, 1970), and I drew great benefit from it.

Imagery has a way of emphasizing to a person that they are more powerful than they thought—the ability to imagine is empowering. Things that can be visualized and practiced in imagination may well lose much of their power to create anxiety. The ability of the mind to symbolize and thus to separate from being completely merged with the imagined thing, person, or situation is one of the most powerful resources that we can learn through therapy. It is a property of a mature mind that many ignored children have never been taught and that may well be a major deficit in their development. Imagination also enables us to control our own feeling states by conjuring up powerful images of safety, courage, happiness, warmth, being accepted, and so on. A terrifying task can become an exciting adventure if our mind is able to find the images that cue such thoughts and feelings.

Images have the particularly useful property of being half involuntary (they happen while the client watches) and half voluntary (clients can essentially visualize whatever they want), rather like transitional objects (Winnicott, 1971). Moreover, the therapist can make very simple interventions that open the client's mind to new possibilities ("Look around you: perhaps you can see an opening in the wall that surrounds you"). As a result of this, images happen in a transitional space, and the broadening of this transitional space can be enormously healing for clients who have been ignored children; images can foster an inner spaciousness and an ability to influence the world in ways of which many anxiety-ridden clients have not previously dreamed.

The space in which imagery takes place, this curious borderland between the reflective and the spontaneous, has features of an altered state of consciousness and has also been called a "liminal" space (Schwartz-Salant, 1989). The concept of liminality is often applied to processes of learning and is therefore relevant for psychotherapy. It describes the state of confusion and disorganization that precedes new *knowing* and forms the middle phase (the phase of "not knowing") of a learning process. Using imagery, it is often possible to hold a client in a liminal state for some time. In this state, thoughts and feelings have a particularly fluid quality that opens the possibility of deep change in a very stuck situation. In rituals, we often visit liminal spaces, and therapy with images can resemble rituals during which a new state of being arises in our imagination and has a chance to grow and solidify in the imaginary world before percolating gradually into everyday consciousness.

In the first few years of our lives, our brains are full of furiously sprouting neurons that want to make tens of thousands of connections with other neurons. Learning how to be in the world requires the brain to select a subset of these connections and networks and strengthen them, while pruning out connections and networks that are not being used. The rate at which new neurons arise in the brain and the rate at which they sprout and create new connections both slow down considerably after the first few years of life, as the main pathways and networks that we build our identity around get more defined. After that, we can no longer rely on our brains being able to establish new pathways with the ease and speed of our early childhood. If our early childhood has involved developmental deficits, we can assume our brains to be poorer in the number of pathways and networks that we have available. It seems to me that as adults, we have to deliberately promote the activation of new pathways and networks in our brains if we want to fill in some of these deficits. Our imagination is a way of switching on brain capacities and domains that we have not hitherto made use of and, in the case of many ignored children, even have been a bit fearful of.

Fantasies; daydreams; visualizations; dream interpretations; or improvised play involving creative arts, movement, or any other media: these are the best ways we have to create the material that can fill in our developmental deficits. Many ignored children are avid readers and use stories to fulfil this role. Others like music or painting or play very physical games. Some write poetry or books. In addition, therapeutic interventions that deliberately create inspiration are important steps toward the filling in of developmental deficits.

Over the years I have learned to keep an eye out for anything that resembles an image that the client brings spontaneously. Every time a client uses a metaphor to describe an inner state of their mind, they are giving us a present that we can make use of in order to help them elaborate further, thus breathing more life into it. There are also a variety of ways to encourage clients to deliberately create images in their minds. For some clients using body sensation as a starting point works really well. Others like to use physical means such as toys or buttons to set up an image. Others like visual materials such as postcards or bring their own dreams to therapy. Some find it enough to relax and close their eyes to gain access to inner images.

I have already commented on the possibility of processing imagined targets in EMDR. Sometimes these arise as typical scenarios in which the client has no specific memory of a defined event but has a clear image that illustrates the issue that we are trying to process. I tend to treat them in much the same way that I would treat real memories of single events. Often just setting up such targets is therapeutic, in that it gives clients a place to put their distress that is different from the endless and fruitless ruminations they are used to. An image evokes the possibility of something new happening and sets the scene for change. Of necessity, the processing of such targets then becomes an imaginary journey and can take clients to unexpected and new places. Care needs to be taken with clients who tend to use imagery to avoid coming to terms with the real world. Those ignored children who start out being unable to see beyond their own suffering can benefit enormously from a more playful and creative way of relating to their own life stories and from a realization that they themselves have far more resources available to change their lives than they ever thought.

The specific imaginal approaches available to psychotherapists are many, and only a few of them are known to me. I have learned from psychosynthesis, transpersonal psychotherapy, and Jungian analysis, as well as the more psychoanalytically inspired Katathymes Bilderleben (an imaginal approach derived from psychoanalysis and in wide use in the German-speaking part of the world) and some approaches derived from energetic healing and shamanism. No doubt readers will find other sources or create their own according to the needs of any individual client.

Towards the end of his therapy, Norman spends several sessions debating with himself whether to remain living where he is or whether to move back to the town where he grew up. Noticing that rational arguing back and forth doesn't resolve the dilemma, I suggest trying a different approach and, after instructing him on how to relax, ask him to visualize walking down a path that forks after a while. I ask him to imagine two signposts with the names of the places under consideration on them. I suggest he look at the place where the path branches closely and then walk along one branch of it, observing how it looks, what he encounters, how he feels walking along this path, and where it leads. Then I ask him to do the same with the other branch.

Throughout the exercise, Norman reports strikingly detailed and vivid images back to me. He sees the place where the path branches as a dark wood with rocks on both sides of the path and deep drifts of dead leaves underfoot. The first branch he explores is signposted to his childhood home. He almost immediately starts to encounter animals, squirrels, a cat, birds. The terrain soon opens out and he emerges into a sunlit landscape that feels calm and welcoming to him. Going back, he explores the second branch signposted to his current home. This path continues much the same as the path he has come by. After some time, the wood comes to an end here too, but the landscape he encounters has a much bleaker look to it and does not feel comfortable or welcoming at all.

When he opens his eyes after the exercise, he is stunned by how clear his decision appears on this imaginary level. I can see what a great relief it is for him to have contacted the place inside that is able to make this decision in a way that feels right.

He talks about this exercise again a few weeks later and tells me that he is interested to explore this newfound source of wisdom inside more. He especially wonders if it could help him come to terms with the loss of a mother that he can't really remember.

I take him on another imaginary journey, along another path, and ask him to imagine coming to a house where a mother lives and meeting this mother. It takes him quite a long time to find such a house. The countryside that his path leads him through seems uninhabited. I keep telling him to go on, through rocky terrain and then across a river on precarious stepping stones. In the middle of the river, he feels like giving up. I tell him to take a deep breath and feel his feet standing firm on the stones. He manages to go on and reach the other side—and there is the house. As he approaches it, he is immediately able to visualize the mother who emerges from it. He feels a bond with her from the beginning, and is able to imagine her speaking to him in kind and loving words, reaching out to him, touching him, and inviting him to spend time with her. The following week, he reports that he has felt quite content in his own company, secure in the knowledge that he can imagine having the mother he needed as a child any time. The richness of the images he is able to visualize helps him enormously to have a sense that he is finding inside himself what he lost early in life.

Concluding Remarks

I want briefly to go back to where I started this book, to the description of a typical person who was an ignored child. I have hitherto depicted the more problematic characteristics of such a person, the characteristics that they or others decide require the attention of a psychotherapist. I feel it is important also to highlight those of their characteristics that are valuable resources both for the individual and for the wider world. For me as a psychotherapist it has always been important to see the traits of my clients that make me love them and admire them and that are a source of inspiration for me.

If we are to support ignored children in their therapeutic process, we need to appreciate the adaptiveness of their coping strategies and some of the precious qualities that derive from them. Some of these qualities are loyalty, consideration of others, cooperativity, humility, diligence, persistence, self-reflectiveness, a willingness to take responsibility for themselves, and a love of peace. If you are looking for a person who takes their job seriously and will do their utmost to carry it out it properly, you want an ignored child. The same applies if you need a person to sustain and nurture those in need of sustaining and nurturing, or if you need a person who can be patient and dutiful, or a person who is capable of putting themselves in the service of a greater cause.

It seems obvious to me that ignored children possess to a great degree the qualities that keep most families and societal institutions functioning, even if they do not take on flamboyant leadership roles and might find those on the whole too stressful. For roles that mean working quietly in the background, perhaps as part of a team, and keeping the show on the road, we cannot do better than to trust ignored children. Most of us benefit in some way from having ignored children around to provide support and help when we need it. Many of us view loyal service as somehow less valuable than leadership, but in order for there to be a functioning society, there is a need for both, and both are of equal value (Cain, 2012).

However, the experience of most ignored children is a very different one. What they see is that the world privileges extroversion over introversion, self-promotion skills over competence and diligence, leadership qualities over teamwork, and having fun over fulfilling one's duties. In such a world, they generally do not feel valued and may instead feel overlooked, dismissed, or ridiculed. Perhaps we should not be surprised that the value of ignored children to society is being ignored just as they are themselves.

The experience of being undervalued and dismissed starts in childhood. Emotionally neglected children typically think and behave in ways that current Western society does not encourage. Western society likes children who are boisterous, confident, gregarious, popular, adventurous, and eager to shine. Once they are grown up, being extroverted, confident, independent, entrepreneurial, and ambitious is still encouraged, admired, and rewarded.

It is easy to see from this that clients who were ignored children are very nearly the opposite of what is seen as desirable. Instead of boisterous, they are quiet and retiring; instead of confident, they are anxious and compliant; instead of gregarious, they are shy; instead of extroverted, they are introverted; instead of popular, they are nerdy loners;

instead of adventurous, they are diligent; and instead of eager to shine, they are ashamed of themselves and want to hide.

Such experiences can lead to a sense of being on the margins of mainstream culture or even being part of a minority that is discriminated against. Such feelings cannot be kept out of the therapy room and will be part not only of our clients' life stories but also of the therapeutic relationship.

In the therapy of ignored children, we often encounter clients who feel taken advantage of, dismissed, misunderstood, and exploited by others, whether that be in the workplace or in families. This position in their social environment causes much stress, heartbreak, and powerless frustration to adults who were ignored children. Moreover, individuals who were ignored children are typically not well equipped to deal with these difficulties: they generally find asserting themselves and setting boundaries arduous if not impossible and will be most hesitant to walk away from exploitative relationships. This will need to be addressed in the therapy.

The fact is that people with the characteristics of ignored children have lower social rank than those who conform better to the prevalent societal value system. As such, they have to expect to experience more stress than those in positions of higher social rank (see for example Adler et al., 2000). We have to remember that this additional stress comes on top of all the stresses that ignored children already experience as a result of their developmental difficulties and deficits.

It will be necessary in therapy both to acknowledge this injustice and the fact that the client does not deserve such bad treatment. It will also be advisable to work toward shifting the locus of control of their self-esteem to an internal place, where they are not overly affected by other people's judgments but can maintain their own sense of worth. If they manage to do this to the point where they take it for granted that they are acceptable, they may well find a higher degree of acceptance by the world around them (Stauffer, 2004).

The increasing polarization between those in power and the disempowered in current Western society thus comes directly into the therapy room, in a way that can be viscerally experienced by both therapists and clients. Therapists may act out the dynamic unconsciously by not taking their clients who were ignored children very seriously and by taking advantage of their compliance and politeness. Alternatively, they may be pushed toward rebelling against the prevalent culture that risks oppressing more and more individuals who deviate, even a little, from the expected norm. It may also lead clients to actively seek out individuals and groups that are more congenial and supportive of their own ways of being, and this can potentially be a very empowering experience for these clients.

The potential for political activism is not the only relevant aspect of the neglect of neglect by our society. The expectations and value systems of the society in which we live are inevitably internalized. Tacit expectations on how we should be, as well as prevalent moral and ethical judgments and beliefs, cultural norms, and religious beliefs and attitudes all shape our thinking, including our thinking about ourselves. These internalized judgments will come into the therapy room as negative introjects, causing clients feelings of shame and persistent self-criticism.

We can thus expect our clients to have powerful, internalized judgments about the very same characteristics that make them valuable members of society. For clients who were ignored children, the shame and feeling of inferiority relating to the coping strategies that they have learned through being ignored children adds considerably to the burden of their suffering. Clients who were ignored children will typically feel unacceptable by mainstream society, and this may engender feelings of anger, resentment, and hatred, or shame, despair, and hope-lessness. These may take up a lot of space in the therapeutic process, and it will be important for the therapist to be able to help their client work through the issues related to how damaging and life-limiting such introjects can be.

Of course, therapists live in the same society and therefore have these same introjects. Even if most therapists probably have a narra-tive of themselves as champions of the oppressed, there may be dilem-mas for therapists who would like for their clients to become more acceptable in mainstream society but also to be allowed to be them-selves, without the stigma of pathology where there shouldn't be one. Such dilemmas need to be held in mind and probably worked through by therapists themselves.

Therapists of clients who were ignored children will need to reex-amine their own beliefs and assumptions about what is desirable in a human life. If a client chooses to forego ambition for the sake of sup-portive contact within a team where they can disappear a little into the background, can we support them in this aim without reservation? Or if a client expresses a wish to minimize human contact in their life, will we refrain from trying to nudge them toward a more active social life? What about the client who avoids arguments with their family members—can we relinquish our judgment about the benefit of clients expressing their authentic feelings?

I have often found it necessary to review some of my own preconcep-tions around what good therapy should aim for and have found this to be helpful in the therapy of ignored children. While bearing in mind what philosophy, statistics, and biological sciences teach us about what a good life ought to be, for those individuals who were ignored chil-dren it may be much more helpful to strike a balance between this and what is actually possible and comfortable for them. I believe that discussing the striking of such a balance in a dispassionate way models an approach to life that is not under the iron control of rigid and fear-based or shame-based judgments, but that allows space for thinking about how we want to live. In turn, this allows the reexamination of our values in the light of experience and helps create an inner therapist to help us adapt to changing circumstances.

At the end of the day, what I have just outlined challenges the clients' ability to come to terms with the limitations of their own lives and with the injustice of the world in which they live. I find the process of realizing and accepting that there may be limits to the size and shape of the life that is possible for a client who was an ignored child is a long and painful one. It may include coming to terms with being unable to hold down a long-term relationship, have children, be successful professionally or politically, earn a lot of money, and live an affluent lifestyle. There will be other unpalatable and limiting aspects of a person's existence that may have to be accepted. As in most psychotherapeutic processes, the working through of disappointment will be of central importance. It remains one of the most worthwhile endeavors of psychotherapy.

It now remains to conclude the therapeutic journeys of my four clients:

At the end of 3 years of therapy, **Mortimer** has managed to move to a new job where he has better career prospects and can develop his creativity a bit more. He is satisfied with where he is heading professionally and indeed gets a lot of praise for his intelligence and the creative solutions he finds for problems. Sadly, his girlfriend has left him, saying she felt too bored with him, and this has taken a lot of time for him to come to terms with. However, he has managed to separate from her and in the process has also separated quite a bit from his parents, so that on the whole he is much more his own person. Going through the separation from his girlfriend has also changed his relationship with anxiety, and he says now, "I don't have very much to fear these days—bad things have happened, and I have survived them, and that puts fear into perspective."

I am amazed when I look at him now. Instead of seeing a boy hunched under the burden of his life, with a pale, pinched face and a tendency to make himself invisible, these days I see a young man who fills his body, stands up much straighter, and seems to have grown in every way. Each time he enters my therapy room, I am slightly surprised at how much taller he is than I have remembered. His face is softer yet has lost the childlike, pleading look. He has experienced hardship and come through it and has matured along the way. With his own gentle sense of humor, he does not hesitate to poke fun at me occasionally, and I feel delighted that my more parental stance gets kindly but firmly put into place as he practices his stronger boundaries on me.

He has formed some good friendships with work colleagues and most recently has met another young woman who sounds like she could be a much kinder version of the previous girlfriend. He ends therapy shortly after the new girlfriend moves in with him, and he goes off feeling that he is much better equipped now to face the world and be in charge of his own life.

Norman has been in therapy with me for 6 years when he retires from work and decides to move back to the town where he grew up. He feels that it will be easier for him to reactivate childhood friends and relations rather than to try and form new close relationships here. He describes himself as much less depressed—in fact he very rarely feels the old despair and despondency now. He says he feels softer than before and more alive and more able to be grateful for the good things in his life.

I can see the increased aliveness in his eyes. Instead of looking rather withdrawn and inward-looking, they are now awake and engaged with his surroundings. Along with his ability to visualize situations that make him feel good, a whole host of new resources has surfaced. For example, he has rented a plot in a community garden and now spends quite a bit of time there, enjoying the work and the companionship with like-minded neighbors. He also sings again regularly although he has not wanted to rejoin a choir; that will be a project for life in his new home.

Ending his therapy is a big deal for both of us, because of how deeply he has been attached to me. There are numerous memories of misattuned, shaming, and hurtful incidents in sessions to be narrated, understood, apologized for, and forgiven. This process takes several sessions. It helps him to be able to say what wasn't okay and to be heard in that pain. For me, these sessions are also an important learning experience. In addition, I become aware of what a big part of my working life he has been and how much such a faithful client who turned up regularly has contributed to stability in my life. I do what I can to enable him to take feeling valuable and lovable with him into his new life.

I hear from him after 6 months to say that he is well settled in and feels the move has been worthwhile as he has found a sense of belonging with a circle of good friends. He happily tells me of all the activities that he has initiated in order to make his retirement enjoyable and still feel that he contributes something of value to the community in which he lives.

Olivia has done very well with the early trauma EMDR approach and reports a massive change in her baseline state. "I've gone from being mostly anxious and trying very hard not to make mistakes, to being much more relaxed and secure, enjoying myself even." She is still struggling with her new relationship. There are many things "wrong" with her new partner, and he also finds many things "wrong" with her, and so they both are having to learn what to do with their mutual disappointment in each other. At one point, they decide to separate and live apart for several weeks. Then they both realize that actually what they gain from being together far outweighs the difficulties, and so they get back together.

Olivia remains in therapy for a very long time—there is so much to work through, especially her childhood with her very difficult adopted mother and all her struggles in early adulthood. She ends therapy as she, too, reaches retirement, after nearly 10 years of therapy, and as she prepares to enjoy a more leisurely pace of life with her partner. "We will live on a fairly small budget, but I feel so strongly that we have both deserved some good times."

I look back at how she was when we started and can see a very great difference. It seems as if the essential person that she is used to be grayed over with anxiety and shame, and it is now more clearly visible. No longer does she give the impression of a person who has to work hard to appear normal; instead, she is comfortable with herself and, while still rather shy, does not seem to be so crippled with shame any more. Instead the basic comfort with being who she is shows in her face and in the posture and movements of her body. I find the way she has accepted the many limitations to her life a true inspiration, and together we can appreciate how much this has transformed her personality. She has gone from a very superego-driven and compliant person to somebody who has found contentment in inhabiting both her shortcomings and her resources. She ends on a note full of confidence in her ability to create a good life for herself.

Pearl decides to end her therapy after about 5 years, a year after her daughter has moved away to a university. Pearl is very happy with how her daughter has developed and how much easier their relationship has become. The key to this was understanding that her daughter was taking sides in a conflict that had always been inside Pearl herself and was therefore throwing her fragile internal equilibrium into chaos.

She is still struggling to set boundaries in her work as a school teacher. We have come to realize that a school is a being with bottomless needs, and nobody can fulfil them all. In order to survive being in a school, everybody has to learn to put some boundaries into place—but this may always remain a challenge for Pearl. The thing that has really changed for her is that her caregiving is not so one-sided and not so compulsive and panic-driven. Instead, she comes across as a very loving and bighearted person with a lot to give.

Her decision to end therapy starts to form after a birthday party that her husband and her children arrange for her as a surprise. She experiences an outpouring of love from her immediate family that she has never felt before, and it makes her feel completely happy and think that she really has everything she has ever wished for. "It has been a long way from when we first said that I needed to find more balance in my relationships, so that those who wanted my love also had to give me theirs. Back then I was terrified to make such an outrageous claim on other people. But now it feels like that has come true, and I am so happy!"

She knows that this state of happiness will not be constant. Her mother is still alive and still as envious as ever, and there are always moments when old insecurities and old destructive impulses claw at her. But the power of her mother's envy has been broken, and Pearl has an equal power to set against it in the love and satisfaction she feels in her work as a teacher and in her role as a mother and wife.

As we are about to end, I tell her how much love radiates from her face, and how few people I have known who are able to give so much and so freely. She blushes slightly and then says: "Yes, it's true. I find mostly these days that I can give from a place in my heart where there is real abundance, and as long as I can keep in contact with this place, giving to others nourishes me, too."

Acknowledgments

I owe a huge debt of gratitude to Babette Rothschild, who has supported me throughout in writing this and emphasized how important it was for this book to exist. I am indebted to John Waterston, John Henry, and the members of my peer supervision group for their contributions. Deborah Malmud has believed in my book, and my gratitude to her is enormous. I also want to thank the editorial team at Norton for their uncountable excellent suggestions. A special thank you goes to all my friends and colleagues who have made contributions to this work: Jill van der Aa, Merete Holm Brantbjerg, Lynne Holmes, Elfriede Kastenberger, and Sofia Petridou. My other friends and family members have supported and encouraged me. All my supervisees have inspired my work and contributed their thinking and in some cases, their client stories. And last not least, I thank from the bottom of my heart all my wonderful clients, without whom I would know nothing and would not have been able to write this book.

References

Adler, N. E., Epel, E. S., Castellazzo, G., & Ickovics, J. R. (2000). Relationship of subjective and objective social status with psychological and physiological functioning: Preliminary data in healthy, White women. *Health Psychology, 19*(6), 586–592.

Ainsworth, M. D. S., Blehar, M., Waters, E., & Wall, S. (1978). *Patterns of attachment.* Hillsdale, NJ: Erlbaum.

Alexander, F. (1950). *Psychosomatic Medicine.* New York: W.W. Norton.

Allin, H., Wathen, C. N., MacMillan, H. (2005). Treatment of child neglect: A systematic review. *Can. J. Psychiatry, 50*(8), 497–504.

Assagioli, R. (1999). *Psychosynthesis: a manual of principles and techniques.* London: Thorsons.

Beebe, B., & Lachmann, F. (2002). *Infant research and adult treatment: Co-constructing interactions.* Hillsdale, NJ: Analytic Press.

Berntson, C. G., Cacioppo, J. T., Quigley, K. S., & Fabro, V. T. (1994). Autonomic space and psychophysiologcal response. *Psychophysiology, 31*(1), 44–61.

Boadella, D. (1987). *Lifestreams.* Hove, UK: Routledge.

Bogdan, R., Williamson, D. E., & Hariri, A. R. (2012). Mineralocorticoid receptor Iso /Val (rs5522) genotype moderates the association between previous childhood emotional neglect and amygdala reactivity. *Am. J. Psychiatry, 169*, 515–522.

Bowlby, J. (1951). Maternal care and mental health. *Bull World Health Organ, 3*(3), 355–533.

Bowlby, J. (1969). *Attachment and loss. Vol. 1: Attachment.* New York: Basic Books.

Bowlby, J. (1973). *Attachment and loss. Vol. 3: Loss.* New York: Basic Books.

Boyesen, G. (Ed.) (1980). *Collected papers on biodynamic psychology.* London: Biodynamic Psychology Publications.

Boyesen, G. (1987). *Über den Körper die Seele heilen* [Healing the soul through the body]. Munich: Kösel.

Boyesen, G., & Bergholz, P. (2003). *Dein Bauch ist klüger als du* [Your belly is cleverer than you]. Hamburg: Miko-Edition.

Brown, W. (2014). *Emotional abuse and neglect of children.* York, PA: William Gladden Foundation Press.

Bullington, J., Nordemar, R., Nordemar, K., & Sjöström-Flanagan, C. (2003). Meaning out of chaos: A way to understand chronic pain. *Scand. J. Caring Sci., 17*(4), 325–331.

Cain, S. (2012). *Quiet: the power of introverts in a world that can't stop talking.* New York: Random House.

Carroll, R. (2001). The autonomic nervous system: barometer of emotional intensity and internal conflict. Retrieved June 16, 2009, from http://www .thinkbody.co.uk/papers/autonomic-nervous-system.htm.

Carroll, R. (2002a). Biodynamic massage in psychotherapy: Re-integrating, re-owning and re-associating through the body. In T. Staunton (Ed), *Body psychotherapy* (pp. 78–100). Hove, UK: Routledge.

Carroll, R. (2002b). Why psychosomatisation is complex: Going beyond cause-effect. Retrieved July 12, 2009, from www.thinkbody.co.uk/body-psych/psychosomatisation.htm.

Carroll, R. (2005). Neuroscience and the "law of the self": The autonomic nervous system updated, re-mapped and in relationship. In N. Totton (Ed.), *New dimensions in body psychotherapy* (pp. 13–29). Maidenhead, UK: Open University Press.

Carroll, R. (2009). Self-regulation—an evolving concept at the heart of body psychotherapy. In L. Hartley (Ed.), *Contemporary body psychotherapy: the Chiron Approach* (pp. 89–105). Hove, UK: Routledge.

Castonguay, L.G. & Hill, C.E. (2012). *Transformation in psychotherapy: Corrective experiences across cognitive behavioural, humanistic, and psychodynamic approaches.* Washington, DC: APA.

Center on the Developing Child at Harvard University (2010). *The foundations of lifelong health are built in early childhood.* http://www.developingchild.harvard.edu

Cimini, G., & Ferri. G. (2012). *Psicopatologia e carattere. L'analisi reichiana. La psicoanalisi nel corpo ed il corpo in psicoanalisi [Psychopathology and character. Psychoanalysis in the body and the body in psychoanalysis. Reichian analysis].* Rome: Alpes Italia.

Clarkson, P. (1995). *The therapeutic relationship.* London: Whurr Publishers.

Cohn, J. F., & Tronick, E. Z. (1983). Three-month-old infants' reaction to simulated maternal depression. *Child Development, 5*(1), 185–193.

Cori, J. L. (2017). *The emotionally absent mother: How to recognize and heal the invisible effects of childhood emotional neglect.* New York: The Experiment.

Cozolino, L. (2002). *The neuroscience of psychotherapy.* New York: W. W. Norton.

Crum, J., Brown, W. L., & Bitterman, M. E. (1951). The effect of partial and delayed reinforcement on resistance to extinction. *Am. J. Psychol., 64*(2), 228–237.

Damasio, A. (1994). *Descartes' error: Emotion, reason, and the human brain.* London: Putnam.

Damasio, A. (2000). *The feeling of what happens.* New York: Vintage.

Darwin, C. (1998). *The expression of emotions in man and animals* (original work published 1872). Oxford: Oxford University Press.

De Bellis, M. D., Keshavan, M. S., Shifflett, H., Iyengar, S., Beers, S. R., Hall, J., & Moritz, G. (2002). Brain structures in pediatric maltreatment-related posttraumatic stress disorder: a sociodemographically matched study. *Biol. Psychiatry, 1:52* (11), 1066–1078.

De Bellis, M. D. (2005). The psychobiology of neglect. *Child Maltreatment, 10*(2), 150–172.

De Bellis, M. D., Hooper, S. R., Spratt, E. G., & Woolley, D. P. (2009). Neuropsychological findings in childhood neglect and their relationships to pediatric PTSD. *Int. Neuropsychol Soc., 15*(6), 868–878.

de Brébisson, G., & Brami, M. (2018). *Comprendre et pratiquer la psychologie biodynamique [Understanding and practicing biodynamic psychology].* Malakoff, FR: Interéditions.

Dethlefsen, T., & Dahlke, R. (1993). *The healing power of illness*. Dorset, UK: Element.

Dwairy, M. A. (2008). Parental inconsistency versus parental authoritarianism: Associations with symptoms of psychological disorders. *Youth and Adolescence, 37*(5), 616–626.

Eiden, B. (1998). The use of touch in psychotherapy. *Self & Society, 25*(2), 6–13.

Eiden, B. (2002). Application of post-Reichian body psychotherapy: A Chiron perspective. In T. Staunton (Ed), *Body psychotherapy* (pp. 27–55). Hove, UK: Routledge.

Emde, R. N., Polak, P. R., & Spitz, R. A. (1965). Anaclitic depression in an infant raised in an institution. *Am. Acad. Child Psychiatry, 4*(4), 545–553.

Ferrucci, P. (1982). *What we may be: The visions and techniques of psychosynthesis*. Winnipeg: Turnstone Press.

Field, T., Figueiredo, B., Hernandez-Reif, M., Diego, M., Deeds, O., & Ascencio, A. (2008). Massage therapy reduces pain in pregnant women, alleviates prenatal depression in both parents and improves their relationships. *Body Mov. Ther., 12*(2), 146–150.

Fonagy, P. (2001). *Attachment theory and psychoanalysis*. London: Karnac.

Forgash, C., & Copley, M. (Eds). (2008). *Healing the heart of trauma and dissociation*. New York: Springer.

Gauthier, L., Stollak, G., Messé, L., & Aronoff, J. (1996). Recall of childhood neglect and physical abuse as differential predictors of current psychological functioning. *Child Abuse & Neglect, 20*(7), 549–559.

Gerhardt, S. (2004). *Why love matters*. Hove, UK: Routledge.

Gibson, L. C. (2015). *Adult children of emotionally immature parents*. Oakland, CA: New Harbinger Publications.

Goodwin, R. D., Hoven, C. W., Murison, R., & Hotopf, M. (2003). Association between childhood physical abuse and gastrointestinal disorders and migraine in adulthood. *Am. J. Public Health, 93*, 1065–1067.

Grannon, R. (2016). *How to stop an emotional flashback*. Kindle edition.

Grassi-Oliveira, R., & Stein, L. M. (2008). PTSD and emotional distress in low-income adults: the burden of neglect. *Child Abuse & Neglect, 32*(12), 1089–1094.

Gratier, M., & Trevarthen, C. (2008). Musical narrative and motives for culture in mother-infant vocal interaction. *Consciousness Studies, 15,* 122–158.

Groddeck, G. (1949). *Exploring the unconscious.* Plymouth, UK: Vision Press.

Hadar, B. (2008). The body of shame in the circle of the group. *Group Analysis, 41*(2), 163–179.

Hart, S. (2008). *Brain, attachment, personality: An introduction to neuroaffective development.* London: Karnac.

Hartley, L. (Ed). (2009). *Contemporary body psychotherapy: The Chiron Approach.* London: Routledge.

Heim, C., Nater, U. M., Maloney, E., Boneva, R., Jones, J. F., & Reeves, W. C. (2009). Childhood trauma and risk for chronic fatigue syndrome. *Arch. Gen. Psychiatry, 66,* 72–80.

Herzog, J. I., & Schmahl, C. (2018). Adverse childhood experiences and the consequences on neurobiological, psychosocial and somatic conditions across the lifespan. *Frontiers in Psychiatry, 9,* Art. 420.

Hildyard, K. L., & Wolfe, D. A. (2002). Child neglect: Developmental issues and outcome. *Child Abuse & Neglect, 26*(6–7), 679–695.

Hobbs, C. J., & Wynne, J. M. (2002). Neglect of neglect. *Paediatrics and Child Health, 12*(2), 144–150.

Holm Brantbjerg, M. (2012). Hyporesponse: The hidden challenge in coping with stress. *Int. J. Body Psychotherapy, 11*(2), 94–118.

Holm Brantbjerg, M. (2020). Widening the map of hypo-states: A methodology to modify muscular hypo-response and support regulation of autonomic nervous system arousal. *Body, Movement & Dance in Psychotherapy, 15*(1), 53–67.

Hopper, E. K., Grossman, F. K., Spinazzola, J., & Zucker, M. (2018). *Treating adult survivors of childhood emotional abuse and neglect: Component-based psychotherapy.* New York: Guilford Press.

Hughes, K., Bellis, M. A., Hardcastle, K. A., Sethi, D., Butchart, A., Mikton, C., Jones, L., & Dunne, M. P. (2017). The effect of multiple adverse childhood experiences on health: A systematic review and meta-analysis. *Lancet Public Health, 2,* e356–e366.

Johnson, S. (1985). *Characterological transformation: The hard work miracle.* New York: W.W. Norton.

Johnson, S. (1994). *Character styles.* New York: W.W. Norton.

Joseph, R. (1999). Environmental influences on neural plasticity, the limbic system, emotional development and attachment: a review. *Child Psychiatry Hum. Dev., 29*(3), 189–208.

Kaufmann, G. (1980). *Shame: The power of caring.* Rochester, VT: Schenkmann Books.

Knight, J. (2008). Loving eyes. In C. Forgash & M. Copley (eds.), *Healing the heart of trauma and dissociation* (pp. 181–225). New York: Springer.

Kulich, R. J., Mencher, P., Bertrand, C., & Maciewicz, R. (2000). Comorbidity of post-traumatic stress disorder and chronic pain: Implications for clinical and forensic assessment. *Curr. Rev. Pain, 4*(1), 36–48.

Landale, M. (2002). The use of imagery in body-oriented psychotherapy. In T. Staunton (Ed.), *Body psychotherapy* (pp. 116–132). Hove, UK: Routledge.

Lapakko, D. (1997). Three cheers for language: A closer examination of a widely cited study of nonverbal communication. *Communication Education, 46*(1), 63–67.

Leeds, A. M. (2012). Developmental pathways to dissociation: Are we forgetting something? *ESTD Newsletter, 3*(1), 4–9.

Leeds, A. M. (2015). *Learning to feel good sharing positive emotion: The Positive Affect Tolerance protocol.* Paper presented to the EMDR UK and Ireland Conference, March 25, 2015.

Leuner, H. (1970). *Katathymes Bilderleben [Catathymic Imagery].* Stuttgart: Thieme.

Levine, P. A. (1997). *Waking the tiger.* Berkeley, CA: North Atlantic Books.

Lim, M. M., & Young, L. J. (2006). Neuropeptidergic regulation of affiliative behaviour and social bonding in animals. *Hormones and Behavior, 50,* 506–517.

Lopez-Duran, N. L., Kuhlman, K. R., George, C., Kovacs, M. (2013). Facial emotion expression recognition by children at familial risk for depression: High risk boys are oversensitive to sadness. *Child Psychol. Psychiatry, 54*(5), 565–574.

Lowen, A. (1971). *The language of the body*. New Jersey: Prentice-Hall.

Maaz, H. J. (2017). *Das falsche Leben: Ursachen und Folgen unserer normopathischen Gesellschaft [False life: Causes and consequences of our normopathic society]*. Munich: C.H. Beck.

Macnaughton, I. (Ed). (2004). *Body, breath and consciousness: A somatics anthology*. Berkeley, CA: North Atlantic Books.

Maheu, F. S., Dozier, M., Guyer, A. E., Mandell, D., Peloso, E., Poeth, K., Jenness, J., Lau, J. Y., Ackerman, J. P., Pine, D. S., Ernst, M. (2010). A preliminary study of medial temporal lobe function in youths with a history of caregiver deprivation and emotional neglect. *Cognitive, Affective, & Behavioral Neuroscience, 10*(1), 34–49.

Main, M. (1985). Attachment: Overview, with implications for clinical work. In S. Goldberg, R. Muir, & J. Kerr (Eds.), *Attachment theory: Social, developmental and clinical perspectives*. Hillsdale, NJ: Analytic Press.

Marcher, L., & Fich, S. (2010). *Body encyclopedia*. Berkley, CA: North Atlantic Books.

Mehrabian, A., & Ferris, S. R. (1967). Inference of attitudes from nonverbal communication in two channels. *Consulting Psychology, 31*(3), 248–252.

Milgrom, J., Gemmill, A.W., Bilszta, J. L., Hayes, B., Barnett, B., Brooks, J., Ericksen, J., Ellwood, D., & Buist, A. (2008). Antenatal risk factors for postnatal depression: a large prospective study. *Affective Disorders, 108*(1–2), 147–157.

Miller, A. (1981). *The drama of the gifted child*. New York: Faber and Faber.

Moaiku, 2019. http://moaiku.dk/moaikuenglish/englishlitterature/articles_pdf/a4/ROST4presenceskills_a4.pdf (accessed 5 August 2019).

Muller, R. T. (2010). *Trauma and the avoidant client: Attachment-based strategies for healing*. New York: W.W. Norton.

Murray, L. (1992). The impact of postnatal depression on infant development. *Child Psychol. Psychiatry, 33*(3), 543–561.

Murray, L., & Cooper, P. J. (1996). The impact of postpartum depression on child development. *Int. Rev. Psychiatry, 8*(1), 55–63.

Nikulina, V., & Widom, C. S. (2013). Child maltreatment and executive functioning in middle adulthood: A prospective examination. *Neuropsychology,* *27*(4), 417–427. doi:10.1037/a0032811.

Nikulina, V., & Widom, C. S. (2014). Do race, neglect, and childhood poverty predict physical health in adulthood? A multilevel prospective analysis. *Child Abuse & Neglect, 38*(3), 414–424.

Norman, R. E., Byambaa, M., De, R., Butchart, A., Scott, J., & Vos, T. (2012). The long-term health consequences of child physical abuse, emotional abuse, and neglect: A systematic review and meta-analysis. *PLOS Medicine, 9*(11), e1001349.

O'Shea, K. (2009). The EMDR early trauma protocol. In Shapiro, R. (Ed.), *EMDR solutions II.* New York: W.W. Norton.

Paulsen, S. L. (2017). *When there are no words: Repairing early trauma and neglect from the Attachment period with EMDR therapy.* Bainbridge Island, WA: Bainbridge Institute for Integrative Psychology.

Perls, F. S., Hefferline, R. F., & Goodman, P. (1951). *Gestalt therapy: Excitement and growth in the human personality.* New York: Julian Press.

Perry, B. D. (2002). Childhood experience and the expression of genetic potential: What childhood neglect tells us about nature and nurture. *Brain & Mind, 3*(1), 79–100.

Pert, C. B. (1999). *The molecules of emotion: Why you feel the way you feel.* New York: Pocket Books.

Pittenger, D. J. (2002). The two paradigms of persistence. *Genet. Soc. Gen. Psychol. Monogr., 128*(3), 237–268.

Porges, S. W. (2001). The polyvagal theory: Phylogenetic substrates of a social nervous system. *Int. J. of Psychophysiology, 42,* 123–146.

Porges, S. W. (2017). Vagal pathways: Portals to compassion. In E. M. Seppälë (Ed.), *The Oxford handbook of compassion science.* Oxford: Oxford University Press.

Powers, A., Ressler, K. J., & Bradley, R. G. (2009). The protective role of friendship on the effects of childhood abuse and depression. *Depression & Anxiety, 26*(1), 46–53.

Reich, W. (1972). *Character analysis* (Original work published 1933). New York: Noonday Press.

Reynolds, J. L. (1997). Post-traumatic stress disorder after childbirth: The phenomenon of traumatic birth. *Can. Med. Assoc., 156*(6), 831–835.

Robertson, J., & Robertson, J. (1989). *Separation and the very young.* London: Free Association.

Rothschild, B. (1995). Defining trauma and shock in body-psychotherapy. *Energy and Character, 26,* 61–65.

Rothschild, B. (2000). *The body remembers.* New York: W. W. Norton.

Rothschild, B. (2004). Applying the brakes. *Psychotherapy Networker Magazine.* January/February. Washington, DC.

Rothschild, B. (2017). *The body remembers, Vol. 2: Revolutionizing trauma treatment.* New York: W. W. Norton.

Rowling, J. K. (1997). *Harry Potter and the philosopher's stone.* London: Bloomsbury.

Sahar, T., Shalev, A. Y., & Porges, S. W. (2001). Vagal modulation of responses to mental challenge in posttraumatic stress disorder. *Biol. Psychiatry, 49*(7), 637–643.

Schimmenti, A. (2012). Unveiling the hidden self: Developmental trauma and pathological shame. *Psychodynamic Practice, 18*(2), 195–211.

Schore, A. N. (1994). *Affect regulation and the origin of the self.* Hillsdale, NJ: Erlbaum.

Schore, A. N. (2003). *Affect regulation and the repair of the self.* New York: W. W. Norton.

Schultz-Venrath, U. (2018). *Mentalizing shame and shamelessness in groups.* Presentation given at the 24th Bowlby Memorial Conference, September 2018, London.

Schwartz-Salant, N. (1989). *Borderline personality: Vision and healing.* Asheville, NC: Chiron Publications.

Sciarrino, N., Hernandez, T. E., & Davidtz, J. (2018). *Understanding child neglect: Biopsychosocial perspectives.* Cham, Switzerland: Springer.

Shapiro, F. (2001). *Eye movement desensitization and reprocessing: Basic principles, protocols, and procedures.* New York: Guilford Press.

Shapiro, R. (2009). Attachment-based depression: Healing the "hunkered-down." In R. Shapiro (Ed.), *EMDR solutions II* (pp. 90–105). New York: W.W. Norton.

Shipman, K., Edwards, A., Brown, A., Swisher, L., & Jennings, E. (2005). Managing emotion in a maltreating context: A pilot study examining child neglect. *Child Abuse & Neglect, 29*(9), 1015–1029.

Siegel, D. (1999). *The developing mind.* New York: Guilford Press.

Southwell, C. (1988). The Gerda Boyesen method: biodynamic therapy. In J. Rowan & W. Dryden (Eds.). *Innovative therapy in Britain* (pp. 178–201). Maidenhead, UK: Open University Press.

Spitz, R. (1965). *The first year of life: A psychoanalytical study of normal and deviant development of object relations.* New York: International University Press.

Staunton, T. (Ed) (2002). *Body psychotherapy.* Hove, UK: Routledge.

Stauffer, K. A. (2004). Cinderella goes to the ball. *AChP Newsletter, 28, 24.* Retrieved June 11, 2019, from http://www.stauffer.co.uk/ Cinderella.html.

Stauffer, K. A. (2005). From wanting to having: The vasomotoric cycle and receptivity. *Association of Holistic Biodynamic Massage Therapists, 8*(1), 7–9. Retrieved July 1, 2009, from http://www.stauffer.co.uk/Receptivity.htm

Stauffer, K. A. (2009). Self-regulation: The ways of nature. *ATTACHMENT: New Directions in Psychotherapy and Relational Psychoanalysis, 3*(1), 30–37.

Stauffer, K. A. (2010). *Anatomy & physiology for psychotherapists: Connecting body & soul.* New York: W. W. Norton.

Stern, D. (1991). *Diary of a baby: What your child sees, feels and experiences.* London: Fontana.

Strathearn, L., Gray, P. H., O'Callaghan, M. J., & Wood, D. O. (2001). Childhood neglect and cognitive development in extremely low birth weight infants: A prospective study. *Paediatrics, 108*(1), 142–151.

Straus, M. A., & Kantor, G. K. (2005). Definition and measurement of neglectful behavior: Some principles and guidelines. *Child Abuse & Neglect, 29,* 19–29.

Taillieu, T. L., Brownridge, D.A., Sareen, J., & Afifi, T. O. (2016). Childhood emotional maltreatment and mental disorders: Results from a nationally representative adult sample from the United States. *Child Abuse & Neglect, 59,* 1–12.

Teicher, M. H., Dumont, N. L., Ito, Y., Vaituzis, C., Giedd, J. N., & Anderson, S. L. (2004). Childhood neglect is associated with reduced corpus callosum area. *Biol. Psychiatry, 56*(2), 80–85.

Totton, N., & Edmondson, E. (1988). *Reichian growth work.* Dorchester, UK: Prism Press.

Trevarthen, C. (1993). The self born in intersubjectivity: The psychology of an infant communicating. In U. Neisser (Ed.), *The perceived self: Ecological and interpersonal sources of self-knowledge.* New York: Cambridge University Press.

Trevarthen, C. (2013). *Embodied wisdom: Intelligence of movement shared from life's beginning.* Presentation given to the Chiron Association for Body Psychotherapists November 2013, London.

Tronick E. (2009, November 30). *Still Face Experiment: Dr. Edward Tronick.* YouTube. https://www.youtube.com/watch?v=apzXGEbZhto&t=86s

Wallin, D. J. (2007). *Attachment in psychotherapy.* New York: Guilford Press.

Weinberg, M. K., Beeghly, M., Olsen, K. L., & Tronick, E. (2008). Effects of maternal depression and panic disorder on mother-infant interactive behaviour in the Face-to-Face Still-Face paradigm. *Infant Mental Health, 29*(5), 472–491.

White, M. (2007). *Maps of narrative practice.* New York: W.W. Norton.

Widom, C. S. (1999). Posttraumatic Stress Disorder in abused and neglected children grown up. *Am. J. Psychiatry, 156,* 1223–1229.

Widom, C. S., Czaja, S., Wilson, H. W., Allwood, M., & Chauhan, P. (2012). Do the long-term consequences of neglect differ for children of different races and ethnic backgrounds? *Child Maltreatment, 18*(1), 42–55.

Winnicott, D. W. (1971). *Playing and reality.* London: Tavistock.

World Health Organization. (2013). *WHO recommendations on postnatal care of the mother and newborn.* Geneva: World Health Organization.

Index

Note: Italicized page locators refer to figures.

absent caregivers, 35, 39, 40 42–44
abuse
  neglect and deleterious effects of, 51
  neglect *vs.,* xiii, 7, 10
  overlap with emotional neglect, 50
  poor health in adulthood and, 119
active interventions, 128
addiction, preoccupied caregivers
  and, 39, 49
adoption, 42, 43, 48
affect regulation, 69, 90
  core sense of self and, 58
  neuroscience of early development
  and, 91–96
agency, 184
aggressor, reframing identification
  with, 160
Alexander technique, 125
alexithymia, 176
allergic reactions, 119
ambivalent attachment style, 56
amygdala, reactive, emotional
  neglect and, xv, 90

anger, oral character style and,
  76–77
ANS. *see* autonomic nervous system
  (ANS)
anxiety, xi–xii, xiv, xv, 1, 2
  addressing in first stage of therapy, 162–63
  developmental deficits and, 27
  ignored children and, xiv
  regulating, 69
archaic (or malignant) shame, 109
asymmetric relationships, insecurely attached clients and, 154
attachment
  co-creation of a narrative and, 181
  prioritized over self-expression,
  151–52
  shame and ruptures in, 109
attachment-based psychotherapy,
  biodynamic massage integrated
  with, 170
attachment ruptures, repairing,
  129–31

attachment styles, four categories
of, 56
attachment theory
avoidant attachment style and,
55–62
four attachment styles distin-
guished in, 56–57
insecure attachment and, 55
parentification and, 61
attention, neglect *vs.*, 36
autobiographical memories, fragmented, 183
autobiographical self, reparative
experience integrated into, 144
autobiographical timeline, coherent, 183
autonomic nervous system (ANS),
90, 96–102, 120
cycle of self-regulation and, 63–64
hypo-states and, 81
low energy in musculature and low
energy in, 87
polyvagal theory and three
branches of, 102–4
psychoeducation about function
of, 181
shame and shutdown in, 111
trauma and, 100–102
two branches of, autonomic space,
and, 97
vasomotoric cycles and, 97–98
autonomic space, multidimensional
nature of, 97
autonomy, enforced, 24
avoidant attachment style, 56–57,
59, 61

attachment theory and, 55–62
compliant "good" children and,
58–59
avoidantly attached, as misunderstood term, 59–60

benevolent therapists, 135
bereavement, 43
Bodynamic Analysis
Copenhagen school of, 170
hypo-responsiveness model in, 81
biodynamic massage, 164, 165–66,
169–70
biodynamic psychotherapy
advantages of, 69–71
disadvantages of, 71
self-regulation cycle in, 62–71, *63*
blame, therapeutic process and,
40–41
Boadella, D., 185
body psychotherapeutic approaches,
161–62, 163, 164–74
advantages of, 166–67
biodynamic massage, 164, 165–66,
169, 170
disadvantages of, 167
frustration of client's needs and,
168
gratification of client's needs and,
169
mitigating danger of, 167
relational trauma therapy, 170–74
vegetotherapy, 164, 165, 169
body psychotherapy, 55. *see also* biodynamic psychotherapy
body sensations, 165

biodynamic work and emphasis
on, 71
co-regulation and, 70
ignored children and fear of, 24,
124
imagery and, 200
trauma approaches and use of,
185–86
borborygmi, biodynamic massage
and, 166
boundary setting, 99–100, 212
Bowlby, J., 55
Boyesen, G., 63
brain
neurons in, 198–99
three concentric layers in, 92
breathing, body psychotherapeutic
approaches and, 166
bullying, 186
burnout, 59, 87, 94, 184
compulsive caregiving and, 31, 32,
61
traumatization of neglect and, xiii

caregivers
absent, 35, 39, 40 42–44
client conversations with, weighing benefits of, 38–39
depressed, 40, 44–46, 111, 114–15,
120
early loss of, 43
emotionally unavailable, 47
inconsistent availability of, 48–49
preoccupied, 35–36, 39–40, 47–50
Still Face experiment with, 45
see also parents

Center of the Developing Child (Harvard University), 120
cerebral cortex, 92
challenges
avoiding confrontations and, 128,
136–41
decreasing sizes of, 146
dosing down and, 145
inappropriate, getting out of stalemates created by, 138–39
character structure, ego defenses
and, 72
character styles, ego defenses and,
71–72
chronic fatigue, adverse childhood
experiences and, 119
chronic illness, ignored children
and, 119, 124, 125
cingulate gyrus, 92
"collapsed oral character," 76, 79
compassion, 55
"compensated oral character," 76, 79
compliance, 11
avoidant attachment style and,
58–59
depressed mothers and history of,
46
compliments, appreciating, 193
compulsive caregiving, 17, 47, 90,
113–18, 135, 179, 212
as adaptive coping mechanism,
30–33
changing, difficulties in, 117–18
compensated oral character and, 79
parentification and, 61
as successful defense, 79

confidence, shame and inhibition
of, 54
conflict, deficit and, 28, 184
containment, safety and, 128, 129–
36
coping styles of ignored children,
12–18
compulsive caregiving, 17, 30–33
making self small, 12–14
numbing self against the pain,
15–16
shame and, 16–17
co-regulation, in biodynamic work,
70
corrective experiences, body psychotherapeutic approaches and,
167–68
cortisol, resistance to, 96
"counterpulsation," 185
countertransference
avoiding challenges or confrontations and, 137
client falling in love with therapist
and, 144
Cozolino, L., 113, 114
creativity, 167, 199

Damasio, A., 65
Darwin, C., 115
daydreams, 199
death of parent, 43–44
deficit, conflict and, 28, 184
deficit filling, 163–64
deficit orientation, 128, 141–45
depressed caregivers, 40, 44–46, 111,
114–15, 120

depression
maternal, 44–46, 111, 114–15, 120
perinatal, 120
postpartum, 44, 111, 115
developmental deficits, 54, 141,
198–99
anxiety and, 27
consequences of, in the psychotherapy, 23–30
creating a narrative and filling in,
182
emotional neglect and, xiii–xiv
hypo-responsiveness and, 81–88
maternal depression and, 45
paucity of resources and, 141
relational trauma therapy and,
170
developmental stages, 53–54
developmental urge, 53
diabetes, 119
disappointment, working through,
208
dismissive attachment style, 56
disorganized attachment style, 56,
57
dissociation, 66, 93, 101, 102, 104,
123
from physical self, 124
schizoid character style and, 73
distress, somatizing, 122–23
dorsal vagal complex (DVC), 102,
103, 104
dosing down, 128
coping with challenges and, 145–
47
illustration of, 84–85

Drama of the Gifted Child, The (Miller), 114
dream interpretations, 199
DVC. *see* dorsal vagal complex (DVC)
dysregulation, 66, 67

early trauma EMDR, 186–87, 188–90, 211
ego defenses, 68
  character structure and, 72
  character styles and, 71–72
Ego State therapy, trauma work combined with, 187–88
Eiden, B., 72
EMDR. *see* eye movement desensitization and reprocessing (EMDR)
emotional (or vasomotoric) cycle, 63
emotional flashbacks, 188
emotionally neglected people, understanding inner world of, 7–12
emotional neglect
  age of child and impact of, 40
  cultural shifts and notions of, 36–37
  defining, xii–xiii
  early, physical illness in adulthood and, 119–25
  hypo-responsiveness and, 81–82
  main consequences of, xiii–xiv
  overlap with other presentations, 50–51
  reactive amygdala and, xv, 90
  therapeutic process for clients with, xi–xii, xv
  use of term in text, 35
  see also ignored children/ignored child clients
emotional self-regulation
  biodynamic psychotherapy and, 62–71
  social engagement system and, 193
  see also self-regulation
emotions, creating constancy and safety around, 137. *see also* feelings
empathy, 55
endorphins, somatization and secretion of, 123
energetic healing, 201
enjoyment, sharing, 196–97
envy
  forms of, 156
  maternal, 118, 213
  siblings and, 156–57
excitatory processes, 97
excitement, ignored children and avoidance of, 93–94, 105–6
external resources, 11
eye contact
  newly born babies and, 7–8
  proto-conversations and, 57
  in psychotherapy, 106
eye movement desensitization and reprocessing (EMDR), 108
  adjusting anxiety levels with, 163
  bilateral stimulation in, 192
  early trauma EMDR, 186–87, 188–90
  processing imagined targets in, 200

eye movement desensitization and reprocessing (EMDR) (*continued*)
  repairing relationship with child self and, 159
  "Reprocessing" stage of, 141

facial expressions, proto-conversations and, 57
falling in love with therapist, ignored children and, 142–44
false self, compulsive caregiving and, 32
fantasies, 199
fear
  of body sensations, 24, 124
  of change, secondary gain narrative around, 29
  in ignored children, 8–9
  see also anxiety; terror
feelings
  images of, 177
  words integrated with, 176–79
  see also emotions; good feelings perceived as threatening
Feldenkrais movement technique, 125
flashbacks
  alarm about body sensations and, 124
  emotional, 188
freezing, 93, 104
Freud, S., 122
fun and playfulness
  parentified children and lack of, 115–16
  in therapy, 196

gestalt therapy, biodynamic massage integrated with, 170
gestures, proto-conversations and, 57
good attachment, early loss of, 157
good feelings, supporting, 162, 190–97
good feelings perceived as threatening, 128, 154–60
  early loss of a good attachment and, 157–58
  envious environments and, 156–57
  environment of poverty and, 155
  internalized persecution and, 157
  potential impediments to working with, 159
"good-quality touch," 71

Hadar, B., 108, 109
healthy neglect, 36
Holm Brantbjerg, M., 81, 84, 170, 173
humanistic therapy, biodynamic massage integrated with, 170
humiliation
  memories of, 186
  shame in therapeutic relationship and, 147–48
  see also shame
hyperarousal, post-traumatic stress and, 100
hyper-responsive muscles, 171, 172
hyper-responsiveness, developmental origin of hypo-responsiveness *vs.*, 82
hypertension, 119
hypertonic muscles, 81, 83

hypnosis, 108

hypo-responsive muscles, 170–71,
171–72

hypo-responsiveness
derivation of term, 81
developmental deficits and, 81–88
relational trauma therapy and, 84

hypo-states, in ignored children,
81–82

hypotonic muscles, 81, 83

identification with the aggressor,
shame and, 148–49

ignored children/ignored child clients, 161
bias of, in recognizing emotions on
faces, 89
burden of shame for, 18–23
coping strategies and qualities of,
203–4
deficit orientation with, 142
developmental deficits in the psychotherapy and, 23–30
empowering experiences for, 206
experience of, 1–7
fear of good feelings and, 190–91
focus on own narrative and, 41
four types of coping styles of,
12–18
hypo-states found in, 81–82
inconsistent parental availability
and, 48–49
lifestyle changes and, 194
model of mind and, 53–55
negative therapeutic reaction and,
154

oral character style and, 77
physical neglect of, 50
schizoid characters and, 73–74
self-accusations among, 179
shame and, 107–13
slightly disembodied quality
about, 124
society and undervaluing of,
204–5
solitary lives of, 190
somatization and, 122–25
state of internal poverty and,
25–26
subjective experience of, 37, 41
use of term for, xii–xiii, 35
vulnerability to life stresses and,
121
see also emotional neglect; individual ignored child client
vignettes; psychotherapeutic
interventions for ignored children clients; psychotherapeutic
theories about ignored children;
psychotherapy for ignored children clients

imagery
body sensations and, 200
broadened transitional spaces
and, 198
special power of, 197

imaginal work, 162, 197–202

imaginary journey, 200, 201–2

imagination, deficit orientation and,
142

imagined targets, real memories vs.,
processing of, 187

immune function impairment, traumatic birth experiences and, 119

"inbreath," 185

inconsistent availability of caretakers, 48–49

inflammatory bowel disease, early emotional neglect and, 119

inhibitory processes, 97

inner child
  client hatred of, 159–60
  forming empathic relationship with, 180
  safety needs of, 132–33

inner critic, attachment to, 22–23

inner therapist, creating, 184, 208

insecure attachment style, 55, 56, 60–61
  difficulty in saying "no" and, 128, 151–54
  emotional neglect and, xiv, 38
  lifelong consequences of, xv
  repairing relational ruptures and, 129
  shame and, 112

integrative therapy, biodynamic massage integrated with, 170

integrity of the self, reassembling work and, 160

internalized judgments, of ignored child clients, 206–7

internalized persecution, 157

internal knots, oral defenses and, 78–79

internal poverty, 25–26

internal resources, 11, 27

interpersonal bonds, underdeveloped, in ignored children, 93

intersectionality, power issues and areas of, 154

intimate relationships, ignored children and, 98–99

invasion, 36

isometric-type muscle-tensing exercises, 84–85

Johnson, S., 72, 74

joyful experiences, ignored children and lack of, 105

Jungian analysis, imaginal approaches and, 200

Jungian therapy, biodynamic massage integrated with, 170

Katathymes Bilderleben imaginal approach, 200

language, as important ego function, 175. *see also* words and language

laughter, 196

Leeds, A., 192

lifestyle changes, ignored children and, 194

liminal space, imagery and, 198

love, resilience and, 121

loving eyes, secure attachment and, 106

Lowen, A., 72

loyalty to self, 41

mainstream culture, ignored children marginalized in, 204–5

making self small coping style, 12–14

maladaptive coping strategies, addressing, 164

malignant regression

corrective experiences and, 168

therapeutically productive regression *vs.*, 144–45

memory(ies)

large gaps in, 183

real, processing of imagined targets *vs.*, 187

traumatic, processing of, 186

mental health issues, preoccupied caregivers and, 39, 49

Miller, A., 114

mirroring

absence of, 45, 46

affect regulation and, 91

attachment bonds and, 57

children of depressed mothers and, 115

reversal of normal process of, 113–14

model of mind, ignored children and, 53–55

Mortimer (ignored child client)

avoiding challenges with, 140

boundary issues for, 99–100

clinical presentation, 1–2

concluding therapeutic journey with, 208–9

depressed mother and, 45–46

diminished fear of criticism, 158–59

dosing down example with, 84–85, 147

hiding shame and, 110

high energy in the ANS and low energy in the musculature, 87

learning to name feelings, 178–79

making himself small coping style of, 12–14

self-regulation difficulties of, 67–68

shame and, 19

therapeutic considerations with, 26–27

mothers, depressed, 44–46, 111, 114–15, 120

motivational muscle, building up, 26

muscles

hyper-responsive, 171, 172

hypo-responsive, 170–71, 171–72

hypotonic *vs.* hypertonic, 81, 83

see also skeletal musculature

narcissism

pathological caretaking and, 113

primary, 114

narcissistic injuries, 107–8

narrative of the client's history, finding, 162, 179–84

negative self-talk, 192

negative therapeutic reaction, 154

neglect

abuse and deleterious effects of, 51

abuse *vs.*, xiii, 7, 10

attention *vs.*, 36

healthy, 36

hidden nature of, 180

physical, 50

poor health in adulthood and, 119

see also emotional neglect

neurons, in brain, 198–99
Neuroscience of Psychotherapy, The
(Cozolino), 113
neurotic conflicts, 54
nonverbal communication, 175
nonverbal experiences, 163
nonverbal signals, in biodynamic
psychotherapy, 70
Norman (ignored child client)
clinical presentation, 2–4
concluding therapeutic journey
with, 209–11
death of mother and, 43–44
disagreement over political perspectives, 152–53
eye contact and, 106–7
falls in love with therapist, 142–44
high energy in musculature and
low energy in the ANS, 87
insecure attachment style and, 60
numbing self against the pain coping style of, 15–16
shame and, 20
visualization exercise with, 201–2
numbing against the pain coping
style, 15–16

Olivia (ignored child client)
absent caregiver and, 42–43
adopted parents and, 42, 43, 48
clinical presentation, 4–5
concluding therapeutic journey
with, 211–12
early trauma EMDR work with,
188–90

exploring layers of shame with,
112–13
growth in sense of embodiment,
125
high energy in the ANS and less
low energy in musculature, 87
history of severe perinatal trauma,
74–75
relational safety needs of, 132–33
relational trauma therapy
vignette, 85–86
shame and coping style of, 16–17,
19
shame in therapeutic relationship
and, 149–50
oral character style, 55, 75–81
"collapsed" and "compensated"
types of, 76, 79
development of, 76
undoing internal knots in client
with, 78–79
orbitofrontal cortex, 92
overstretched sense, body psychotherapy approach and, 65, 66,
68–70, 161
overwhelmed state, conceptualizing,
100–101

parasympathetic nervous system
downgoing phase in self-regulation cycle and, *63*, 64
inhibitory processes and, 97
pleasurable feelings and, 191
polyvagal theory and division of,
102

state of overwhelm and, 101
parentification, 90, 114, 115
    attachment theory and, 61
    intergenerational dynamics in,
        116
parentified children, preoccupied
    caregivers and, 47, 49
parents
    death of, 43
    inconsistent availability of, 48–49
    see also caregivers
pathological caretaking, 113
Pearl (ignored child client)
    avoidant attachment style and, 59
    clinical presentation, 5–7
    compulsive caregiving and, 17, 31,
        79–81
    concluding therapeutic journey
        with, 212–13
    creating a narrative for, 182–83
    fragile quality of third-layer
        defenses for, 94–96
    high energy in the ANS and less
        low energy in musculature, 87
    learning to accept love from oth-
        ers, 118
    preoccupied mother and, 49–50
    presence skills practiced by, 173–
        74
    reframing boundary setting chal-
        lenge for, 138–39
    selfish feelings and, 156
    shame and, 20
    therapeutic considerations with,
        28

using positive feedback exercise
    with, 192–93
perinatal depression, health risks
    linked to, 120
perinatal period, schizoid character
    style and, 72–73, 74
peripheral nervous system, ANS and
    efferent (motor) branch of, 96
physical comforts, ignored children
    and estrangement from, 125
physical environment, of the ther-
    apy, 134–35
physical illness in adulthood, early
    emotional neglect and, 119–25
physical neglect, 50
physical sensations, ignored chil-
    dren and numbing self against,
    124. see also body sensations
physical symptoms of illness,
    ignored children and terror of,
    124
playfulness. see fun and playfulness
pleasurable experiences, psycho-
    physiological state triggered by,
    191
political activism, 206
polyvagal theory
    parentified children and, 115
    social engagement system and, 90,
        102–7
Porges, S., 90, 102, 106
positive feedback exercise, 192–94
postpartum depression ("baby
    blues"), 44, 111, 115
post-traumatic stress, 69

post-traumatic stress disorder (PTSD), somatization and, 122
poverty, 50
power issues, therapeutic relationships and, 154
preoccupied attachment style, 56
preoccupied caregivers, 35–36, 39–40, 47–50
presence skills, 173
preverbal material, biodynamic work and, 71
primal shame, 109
primary narcissism, 114
protective parental figures, imagining, 192
proto-conversations, attachment bonds and, 57
psychoeducation, creation of narrative through, 180–81
psychomotor development, stages in, 82–83
psychosomatic conditions, 10
psychosynthesis, imaginal approaches and, 200
psychotherapeutic interventions for ignored children clients, 161–202
  body therapeutic approaches, 161–62, 164–74
  creating narrative, 162, 179–84
  five stages in, 162–64
  imaginal work, 162, 197–202
  supporting good feelings, 162, 190–97
  trauma therapy approaches, 162, 184–90

words and language, 162, 175–79
psychotherapeutic theories about ignored children, 53–88
  attachment theory and avoidant attachment style, 55–62
  biodynamic psychotherapy and emotional self-regulation, 62–71
  hypo-responsiveness and developmental deficits, 81–88
  model of mind and, 53–55
  oral character style, 55, 75–81
  schizoid character style, 55, 71–75
psychotherapy for ignored children clients, 127–60
  avoiding challenges and confrontations, 128, 136–41
  deficit orientation, 128, 141–45
  dosing down, 128, 145–47
  safety and containment, 128, 129–36
  seven major dos and don'ts in, 128
  shame in the therapeutic relationship, 128, 147–51
  understanding and, 127
  when feeling good becomes threatening, 128, 154–60
  working with insecurely attached clients who cannot say no, 128, 151–54

reactive amygdala, emotional neglect and, xv, 90
reading, imaginal work and, 199
recognition shame, 109
regression, malignant vs. therapeutically productive, 144–45

Reich, W., 72

relational trauma therapy, 84, 170–74

  resource-oriented skills training and, 87–88

  valuable contributions of, 87

  vignette, 85–86

reparative experience, integrating into autobiographical self, 144

reptilian brain, 93

resentment, oral character style and, 76

resilience

  of human psyche, 184

  love and, 121

  see also resources

resistance

  biodynamic work and, 70

  body psychotherapeutic approaches and, 166, 169

  to cortisol, 96

  to therapy, 10–11

resonance, attachment bonds and, 57

resource-oriented skills training, 87–88

resources

  dependence on small number of, 25

  external, 11

  hypo-states and lack of, 82

  internal, 11, 27

  poverty and scarcity of, 155

  somatization and paucity of, 123–24

  utilizing to maximum capacity, 16

re-traumatization, avoiding, 97

reviewing therapy process, 164

rheumatoid arthritis, early emotional neglect and, 119

risk aversion, 25

risk taking, ignored children and, 98

ROST. *see* resource-oriented skills training

Rothschild, B., 174

safety

  aims for, 131

  containment and, 128, 129–36

  fragile sense of, 11

  individualized needs for, 133

  supporting good feelings and, 196

  therapeutic attitudes and interventions around, 134–36

schizoid character style, 55, 71–75, 78

Schore, A., 66, 91

secondary gain hypothesis, 155

secondary gain narrative, around fear of change, 29

secure attachment style

  attachment theory and, 56

  loving eyes and, 106

self-agency, building, 131

self-blaming, 40

self-compassion, 132, 163

self-confidence, 145, 184

self-criticism, 20–22, 24, 206

self-esteem, 16, 17, 20–21, 205

self-expression, attachment prioritized over, 151–52

self-idealization, preoccupied caregivers and, 48
selfishness, exploring beliefs
  around, 156
self-reflection, 92
self-regulation, 92
  ego defenses and, 68
  healthy, 145
  improving, 162–63
  see also emotional self-regulation
self-regulation (or self-regulatory)
  cycles
  in biodynamic psychotherapy,
    62–71, *63*
  embodiment of, 68
  phenomonologic approach to, 70
self-states, Transactional Analysis
  and, 187–88
sexual shame, 109
shadow of sexuality, 109
shallow breathing, 66
shamanism, 201
shame, xii, 5, 10, 90, 107–13, 146
  attachment theory formulation of,
    62
  burden of, 18–23
  coping style tied to, 16–17
  hiding, 110
  inconsistent parental availability
    and, 49
  inhibition of confidence and, 54
  internalized judgments and, 206
  lack of joyful experiences and,
    105–6
  naming, 148

oral character style and, 78
ordinary *vs.* toxic, 107
physical being and, 124
primary function of, 107
resistance to therapeutic change
  and, 23–24
second-generation trauma and,
  111
self-criticism and, 20–22
in the therapeutic relationship,
  147–51
types of, 107–8
in young children, 110–11
shame dimensions, system of, 108–9
shock, polyvagal theory and state of,
  104–5
siblings, envy between, 156–57
silence, in therapy, 134
skeletal musculature
  dorsal vagal complex and, 104
  ego defenses and development of,
    72
  hypo-responsiveness and, 82,
    83–84
  low energy in ANS and low energy
    in, 87
social engagement system, 181
  highly functioning, building, 195
  polyvagal theory and, 90, 102–7
  supporting good feelings and, 193
social environment, marginalization
  of ignored children in, 204–5
social shame, 109
somatic markers, early trauma
  EMDR and, 186

somatization
early emotional neglect and, 119
ignored children and, 122–25
Still Face experiments (Tronick), 45, 180
stillness, polyvagal theory and states of, 102
stress, 51
addressing in first stage of therapy, 162
balance between good care and load of, 121
early neglect, immune function, and, 119, 120
prevalent societal value system and, 205
toxic *vs.* tolerable, 120
traumatic and post-traumatic, 69
stress-management approaches, 163
substance abuse, preoccupied caregivers and, 39, 49
success, importance of, 27
sympathetic nervous system (SNS)
dorsal vagal complex and downregulation of, 103–4
excitatory processes and, 97
safety and low arousal of, 196
state of overwhelm and, 101
upgoing phase in self-regulation cycle and, *63*

terror, 102
about physical symptoms, 124

schizoid character style and, 73, 74
see also anxiety; fear
therapeutic process
active interventions in, 128
slowness of, reasons for, 26–28, 29
therapists
benevolent, 135
clients' falling in love with, 142–44
fun and playfulness with clients and, 196
inner, creating, 184, 208
preconceptions of, reviewing, 207–8
unequal relationship between client and, 154
warmth in, 134
third-layer defenses, fragile quality of, 94–96
tonic immobility, 171
touch
in biodynamic psychotherapy, 71
proto-conversations and, 57
toxic shame, avoiding confrontations and, 136
toxic stress, tolerable stress *vs.*, 120
Transactional Analysis, distinguishing among three self-states of, 187–88
transparency, in therapy, 136
transpersonal psychotherapy, imaginal approaches and, 200
trauma, 54
autonomic nervous system and, 100–102

trauma (*continued*)
  disorganized attachment and, 57
  emotional neglect overlapping
    with, 50
  hypotonic muscle development
    and, 81
  polyvagal theory and, 104–5
trauma therapy approaches, 162,
    163, 184–90
  body sensations used in, 185–86
  early trauma EMDR, 186–87, 188–
    90
  Ego State therapy combined with,
    187–88
  rationale for using, 184–85
traumatic birth experiences,
    impaired immune function and,
    119
traumatic material, body psycho-
    therapeutic approaches and,
    166–67
traumatic shame, 109–10
traumatic stress, 69
Trevarthen, C., 91, 110, 111

Tronick, E., 45, 180
two-chair type techniques, 160

understanding, therapeutic benefit
    of, 127

vasomotoric (or emotional) cycle, 63,
    97–98
vegetotherapy, 164, 165, 169
ventral vagal complex (VVC), 102,
    103, 191
visualization, 197, 199, 201–2
VVC. *see* ventral vagal complex (VVC)

warmth, in therapist, 134
welcoming newly born babies, 7–8
window of tolerance, 87, 97, 120
words and language, 162, 175–79
working alliance, repairing ruptures
    and, 130
"Wounded Healers," 32
writing, imaginal work and, 199

yoga, 125